Phobias
or
The Way of
the Worrier

Phobias
or
The Way of
the Worrier

Tim Weinberg

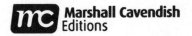
Marshall Cavendish Editions

Copyright © 2010 Tim Weinberg

First published in 2010 by Marshall Cavendish Editions
An imprint of Marshall Cavendish International

PO Box 65829
London EC1P 1NY
United Kingdom

and

1 New Industrial Road
Singapore 536196
genrefsales@sg.marshallcavendish.com
www.marshallcavendish.com/genref

Marshall Cavendish is a trademark of Times Publishing Limited

Other Marshall Cavendish offices: Marshall Cavendish International (Asia) Private Limited, 1 New Industrial Road, Singapore 536196 • Marshall Cavendish Corporation. 99 White Plains Road, Tarrytown NY 10591–9001, USA • Marshall Cavendish International (Thailand) Co Ltd. 253 Asoke, 12th Floor, Sukhumvit 21 Road, Klongtoey Nua, Wattana, Bangkok 10110, Thailand • Marshall Cavendish (Malaysia) Sdn Bhd, Times Subang, Lot 46, Subang Hi-Tech Industrial Park, Batu Tiga, 40000 Shah Alam, Selangor Darul Ehsan, Malaysia

The author and publisher have used their best efforts in preparing this book and disclaim liability arising directly and indirectly from the use and application of this book. All reasonable efforts have been made to obtain necessary copyright permissions. Any omissions or errors are unintentional and will, if brought to the attention of the publisher, be corrected in future printings.

A CIP record for this book is available from the British Library

ISBN 978-1-905736-55-3

Designed and typeset by www.phoenixphotosetting.co.uk

Printed and bound in Great Britain by
CPI Bookmarque, Croydon CR0 4TD

Contents

Introduction

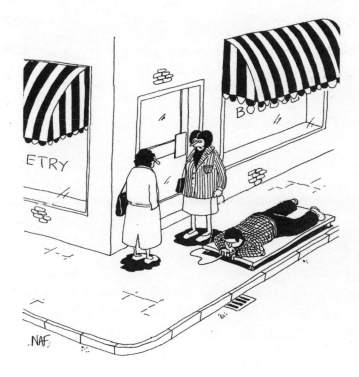

'STEPHEN'S FEAR OF HEIGHTS IS PARTICULARLY BAD TODAY.'

cartoonstock.com

No passion so effectually robs the mind of all its powers of acting and reasoning as fear.

Edmund Burke,
On the Sublime and Beautiful, 1757

Introduction

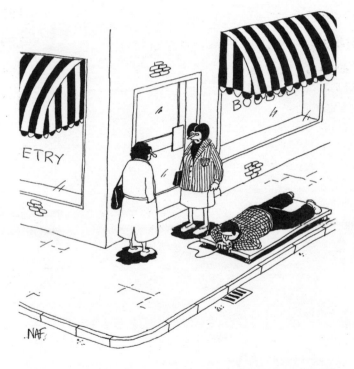

'STEPHEN'S FEAR OF HEIGHTS IS PARTICULARLY BAD TODAY.'

cartoonstock.com

No passion so effectually robs the mind of all its powers of acting and reasoning as fear.

Edmund Burke,
On the Sublime and Beautiful, 1757

What is a phobia?

Let's start with some definitions (and if you are interested in that kind of thing, the sources for all the quotes in the book can be found in the notes at the back):

'Fear, aversion ... unreasoning dislike ... Extreme abnormal fear of, or aversion to, as in acrophobia, claustrophobia.'

'... A very strong irrational fear or hatred of something ... e.g. the place seethed with Europhobia.'

'People with intense, irrational phobias live in perpetual dread of things which would not bother the average person ... some people are even frightened of work itself, while others can get to work and back provided they do not have to travel in rush hour.'

'Aversion, dislike, distaste, dread, fear, hatred, horror, obsession, repulsion, revulsion, terror.'

'A persistent excessive fear attached to an object or a situation that objectively is not a source of danger.'

Got all that? Good. I hope you're taking notes; there will be a test later.

So what exactly is a phobia? Is there more to it than fear? Absolutely. Many people say they are afraid of walking under ladders, for instance. But do they have a phobia? Not necessarily.

Imagine you are walking down the street and you see a ladder leaning against a wall. It's right in your path. You may decide you don't want to walk under it. You may walk around it or even cross the street. But that doesn't mean you have a phobia.

If you did, you would have a much more extreme reaction. On seeing the ladder you would start to feel anxious. As you approached, your breathing would quicken, your heart start to pound, your chest tighten and your mouth go dry. Not only would you go out of your way to avoid the ladder, you would probably avoid ever going near this street again so that you don't run the risk of encountering the ladder a second time or even being reminded of it.

The phobic's lot is to be unable to weigh up a situation that seems entirely innocuous to anyone else. As one expert says, 'anxious individuals inaccurately appraise neutral situations as dangerous .... When [they] are presented with ambiguous scenarios that involve potential harm, they rate negative or catastrophic explanations for the events as being more likely than do non-anxious individuals.'

So simply being scared isn't enough. The word 'phobia' derives from the Greek 'phobos' meaning flight, panic, fear, terror. The Greek god Phobos was said to be so frightening that soldiers painted his face on their shields before battle.

A phobia has two distinct components: the physical and mental turmoil of anxiety and the desire to run away. Aversion and flight together constitute the phobic condition. We're so scared of the consequences of our encounter that even if we flee, we take the terror with us, like the character in Spenser's *Faerie Queen*: 'Still as he fled, his eye was backward cast/As if his fear still followed him behind.'

Perhaps we need philosophy as well as poetry to help us out here. 'The mode of being of fleeing must be explicated by way of the mode of being of fear, or the structures of being which themselves lie in fear.' Enjoy that? Me neither, but don't worry, I won't be talking like that again. It's safe to read on.

Even the names of phobias are confusing, often coupling the Greek suffix 'phobia' with a Latin prefix. This reflects their medical origins but annoys the purists, who like their words to be derived from the Greek or Latin, but not both at once.

Some names for phobias are downright inappropriate. What, for instance, could be more frightening than a fear of space? Answer: a fear for the minds of the cloth-eared simpletons who termed this condition spacephobia. I salute you, Isaac Marks and Paul Bebbington. Great scientists you may be, but you are patently oblivious to the potency and nuance of language, especially when applied to the aberrant and the bizarre.

If a phobia of walking under ladders genuinely existed, I probably wouldn't have used it as an example. There is no name (as yet, anyway) for this condition. It belongs to the order of superstitions rather than phobias.

It's often been said that the British are incredibly superstitious. Take me: I avoid walking under ladders, cross my fingers, touch wood, throw spilt salt over my shoulder, and salute magpies. I don't consider these as fears; I don't even think of myself as being particularly superstitious. Usually I'm not even conscious of these actions; they're merely habitual responses. I've learnt them by watching others around me. That raises an interesting question: are we born with fears and phobias already in place or do we learn them through experience?

In his book *Mastering Phobias;* Richard Stern notes that 'Phobic people have been described as extremely intelligent people behaving stupidly.' I have two problems with this characterisation. First, phobias have no respect for intellect. This statement smacks of the self-justification that leads parents to protest that head lice prefer clean hair to dirty (not true – they really don't care). Second, I prefer 'irrationally' to the more judgmental 'stupidly.' Let's say that phobias make people act irrationally, and leave it at that.

It's not my intention to mock the afflicted – after all, I'm one of them myself – but I think it's fair to point out that phobias cover a broad spectrum. Some are likely to strike a chord with many of us (the dark, the elements, snakes), while at the other end of the scale, some are so minutely specific and seemingly trivial as to seem, well, risible to non-sufferers (my apologies to those who suffer from a phobia of having peanut butter stuck to the roof of their mouth).

But just as the US constitution guarantees that all religions are treated equally whether they date back thousands of years or were made up last week, we can't discriminate between phobias; there is no yard-stick to measure the severity of suffering. We can never know if one person's fear of dogs based on a traumatic childhood incident is more worthy of our sympathy and help than someone else's fear of the colour yellow or the number 8.

Where do they come from?

The origin of phobias is hotly debated. One thing that several experts agree on is that they appear to run in families. According to Dr Angharad Rudkin, 'If mum is slightly anxious socially, even young babies can pick up on it. Babies take their cues from parents even from as young as 10 days.' In the same article, the five most common childhood fears are identified as spiders, the dark, water, monsters under the bed and thunderstorms.

One US study on agoraphobia found that 'patients with phobias tended to have either a parent or a sibling affected (but not both).' Similarly, phobias concerning blood also seem to run in families. Maybe this is only to be expected. A phobia sufferer regaling relatives with anecdotes of dread is likely to elicit more sympathy for a fear of blood and gore than for a fear of buttons, say, and it's easy enough to imagine that traumatised family members might go on to develop a similar sensitivity. Some phobias – those concerning medical procedures, for instance – seem to tap into a deep-rooted vulnerability in all of us. And who isn't afraid of their dentist?

Other phobias may be a throwback to early man's struggle with animals and the elements, perhaps representing an inherited trait that humans have developed over millennia to aid self-preservation. Many phobias are about control, or rather its opposite: the sufferer's fear of powerlessness and lack of control. This can easily develop into a fear of fear itself, or how one might react to fear. The fear of phobias, logically enough, is known as phobophobia.

On that note, perhaps it's time to look to psychology. Freud had a lot to say about fear, as you would expect. One of his famous case studies was of a young man called Hans, who had a fear of horses. Freud's interpretation was that Hans hated his father but could not face up to such unnatural feelings, so he transferred them instead to horses. This allowed him to love his father unconditionally. Another Freudian take on phobia is that 'as young children agoraphobics may have feared abandonment by a cold or non-nurturing mother and the fear has generalised to a fear of abandonment or helplessness.'

So if it's not your dad's fault, it's your mum's. As always, you can blame your parents.

The phobia list

In writing this book, I've drawn extensively on www.phobialist.com, a site that attempts to list all known phobias. Its mission is to collect names for phobias purely for the love of words, without comment or analysis. It features over 500 phobias in a simple alphabetical sequence. The site's founder, Fredd Culbertson, explains: 'It started in a bar one afternoon. We were trying to think of the name of a phobia and couldn't think of it. I looked for it when I got home and started writing down the ones I found … I would add another name whenever I came across it. Pretty soon it was a fairly decent list … I don't remember what phobia name we were looking for that started the list.'

For the record, the site features its own "most wanted" list of phobias that don't yet seem to have an established name:

Feet
Suicide
Toy balloons
Glaciers
Salespeople
Cotton balls and buds
Talking animals
Lists
Bats
Keyboards
Underwear
Driving on a highway
Losing a limb
Midgets and dwarfs.

It's fair to say *The Phobia List* is the most commonly quoted site on the Internet, but two others deserve mention and attention; www.fun-with-words.com and *The Phobia Page* at www.ojohaven.com/fun/phobias. html are both immense labours of love and scholarship. Interesting how both these sites have 'fun' in their names and addresses when phobias are anything but, I have a few of my own, as you'll see later.

At the other extreme, some phobias have multiple names – an indication, perhaps, of how prevalent they are. Cats and thunder and lightning fall into this category. If people don't know the name for a phobia, as phobialist.com points out, they usually make up their own, which is one reason why we end up with so many duplicates.

What I've done here is to group phobias both alpha-betically and by psychological type. I don't think that's been done before, and it helps to shed light on where our anxieties lie. The vast majority of phobias are related to our physical being and emotional states. We may live in an apparently boundless universe, but our fears seldom stray far off a well-beaten path.

In between the chapters on different groups of phobias, I've offered a few glimpses into my own struggles with phobia and attempts to conquer it. I wouldn't claim that my experience is either representative or particu-larly extraordinary, but I hope it will strike at least a few chords with other phobia sufferers, and show you non-sufferers how lucky you are not to be bothered by all this stuff.

Throughout the book I've tried to strike some sort of balance between information and entertainment in looking at what turned out to be a highly charged topic. Think of me as a kind of quizmaster in a pub quiz, and if your nerves get a little shaky, by all means have a drink.

As Hunter S. Thompson once said, 'When the going gets weird, the weird turn pro.'

Episode 1:
My phobia and me

It was January 2008 and I was nervous. I was sitting on a train on the way to London to talk to some publishers about a project that was to culminate in the book you're now reading. They were interested in publishing a book on phobias and as luck would have it, I'd written a cover story for Fortean Times (purveyor of "The world's weirdest news stories") on the fear of clowns or coulrophobia. What I'd thought would be a soft target turned out to be a much richer and more complex subject than I'd ever imagined. I was amazed by readers' reactions too. 'Don't send in the clowns' sparked a debate that dominated the magazine's letters page for months.

But none of that made me feel any better. With the benefit of hindsight, I now recognise the symptoms I experienced on that train journey as a classic phobic response: clammy brow, dry mouth, and sweaty palm.

I wanted to run away – the classic flight reflex – but obviously couldn't. I was scared of my fellow passengers, scared of public embarrassment, scared of failure, and paradoxically just as scared of success. My anxiety seemed to grow as I approached my destination. What if the publisher didn't like my ideas?

At Blackfriars Bridge commuters got on and the carriage became uncomfortably crowded. I looked out of the window and saw the golden cross atop St Paul's Cathedral. I tried to imagine Wren's towering achievement glowering down on a city ravaged by fire, alone and aloof in its majesty. I remembered climbing up there as a child with my dad and brother: the seemingly endless spiralling staircases and spectacular views. But for years my fear of heights – acrophobia, from the Greek word acros meaning pointed or sharp – had been getting worse. The childhood thrill of climbing had given way to fear. I wanted to be able to climb St Paul's Cathedral again.

I made it to my meeting without further ado and talked about the book I hoped to write. I wanted it to be personal. Part of it would be about my own journey through phobia.

Some weeks later, I opened a newspaper and a headline caught my eye: 'I jumped out of plane to cure fear of heights.' The acrophobic in question, Gordon Thomson, described the 'sheer blind terror' of his condition: 'this was no logical, rational fear. There was nothing I could do to stop it. I wasn't scared of falling or hurting myself, it was simply a panic attack that would lock my muscles rigid and have me pouring with sweat.' A chance meeting with a hypnotherapist was the catalyst for his recovery: 'She put me in a sort of relaxed, trance-like state and started going back to my earliest memory of my fear … she went further and further back to what I can only assume must have been some past or previous life memory. That was of being in a plane, during World War I and coming down, seeing the ground rushing up at me.'

I scrunched up the paper and chucked it into the nearest bin. It wasn't that I doubted the story or the therapist's methods, but what I needed was something that addressed the here and now. I didn't have time to address epic themes of life, death and reincarnation.

I thought of another acrophobic's way of dealing with his fear of heights. The French climber Alain 'Spiderman' Robert set out to conquer his vertigo by climbing some of the world's tallest buildings without harness or safety apparatus, at risk of falling to his death at any time. He's clocked up almost a hundred buildings so far, despite accidents that left him severely disabled. What a way to tackle a phobia!

But it wasn't going to be my way.

Self-help and other treatments

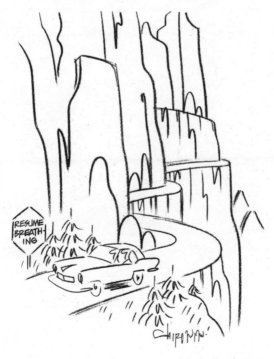

cartoonstock.com

If you're looking for a quick fix, you're in the wrong place. That's not what this book is about.

A health warning

One guide to alternative medicine gives five golden rules to beating phobias on your own:

1. 'Remember that anxiety is unpleasant but seldom harmful.'
2. 'Don't flee from frightening situations.'
3. 'Tell yourself to face up to your fears.'
4. 'The longer you spend confronting your fears, the better you will feel.'
5. 'The sooner you confront your fears, the sooner they will disappear.'

To which I'd add:

6. Ignore all the above until you've read something (*this* thing) on the matter. I reckon the five-point plan might encourage reckless behaviour. When it talks of harm it does so in a strictly physical sense with no concern for psychological damage. It's all very British and stiff upper lip, but I doubt if it has much practical value for phobia sufferers.

Any attempt to tackle a phobia must start with a close look at whatever it is that triggers our anxieties, but I know from experience how difficult it is to get at the root of our fears. It's as though phobias spontaneously spring out of nowhere on some long-forgotten day and stick around forever. I believe you can't hope to isolate these pivotal moments in your life until you start some sort of therapy that will stir up your mind and allow insights to be gleaned.

As one phobia expert says, 'the anxiety sufferer ... cannot always pinpoint the source of his anxiety. And even if he can identify the cause, he cannot avoid encountering it; either the demands of his life situation force him to confront the feared circumstance, or he has so completely internalised his fear that the source of it is within himself.'

I'm aiming to make this book a little more compassionate than the five-point plan. Phobia sufferers aren't faced with the stark choice of pulling themselves together or carrying on suffering; there are various forms of treatment they can seek. Let's take a look at some of them.

Cognitive therapy

Possibly one of the most widely used techniques today, cognitive therapy is associated with Dr Aaron Beck, whose influence must loom large over any book on the topic of phobias. Using 'problem-solving techniques to correct distortions of thinking based on mistaken beliefs,' Beck initially focused on treating depression before applying his techniques to phobias. The therapist focuses on the patient's perspectives, internal logic and self-awareness and tries to rationalise and reduce the disproportionate anxiety generated by a phobia.

Beck formulated ten principles for cognitive therapy, which he saw as a complete system of psychotherapy with a distinct therapeutic approach:

1. 'Cognitive therapy is based on the cognitive models of emotional disorders.'
2. 'Cognitive therapy is brief and time-limited.'
3. 'A sound therapeutic relationship is a necessary condition for effective cognitive therapy.'
4. 'Therapy is a collaborative effort between therapist and patient.'
5. 'Cognitive therapy uses primarily the Socratic method.'
6. 'Cognitive therapy is structured and directive.'

7. 'Cognitive therapy is problem-oriented.'
8. 'Cognitive therapy is based on an educational model.'
9. 'The theory and techniques of cognitive therapy rely on the inductive method.'
10. 'Homework is a central feature of cognitive therapy.'

Being aware of one's own thinking is of key importance in cognitive therapy. Patients are asked to be mindful of 'thinking errors' such as exaggerating, 'catastrophizing,' overgeneralizing and ignoring the positive. They have to keep records of their experiences, thoughts and potential strategies for dealing with their phobia.

Beck uses the acronym AWARE to remind patients how to deal with anxiety:

'Accept the anxiety.'
'Watch your anxiety, try to detach from the experience.'
'Act with the anxiety; try to control your breathing.'
'Repeat the previous three steps until your anxiety recedes to a comfortable level.'
'Expect the best, the worst-case scenarios of our fears rarely ever happen.'

Sensational claims are sometimes made for the efficacy of cognitive therapy, but it does seem to be successful in helping a lot of people. Perhaps that's because it appears to be rooted in common sense. Free from the abstract symbolism of Jungian therapy and the free association of Freudian psychoanalysis, it's also reassuringly practical.

Exposure treatment

In this form of treatment, the phobia sufferer is slowly introduced to the thing they fear (or a safer version of it) in a controlled setting. The thinking is that they should realise they're in no real danger and so their anxiety and desire to flee should subside.

There are two drawbacks with this treatment. First, some people can't face any direct contact with the object of their fears, however controlled the environment. Second, this is a slow, gradual process and may require the phobia sufferer to lead an almost hermit-like existence during treatment so as to avoid confronting their phobia in an 'unsafe' (unmediated) environment.

The most intensive form of exposure treatment is called flooding. Here, direct and sometimes extreme contact with the phobia unleashes a tidal wave of fear, which is then supposed to ebb away. In one TV documentary (I can only dimly remember and can't track down), a woman who was scared of cars was stuck in an old banger in the middle of a stock-car race while other cars deliberately smashed into her. My, she certainly faced her fears that day. She screamed a lot and ended up looking utterly traumatised. Cured? I doubt it.

Systematic desensitization

Similar to 'classical conditioning therapy', think 'Pavlov's (salivating) dog', systematic desensitization was developed by psychiatrist Joseph Wolpe, specifically to help in the treatment of phobias and other anxiety disorders. Also known as 'graduated exposure therapy' its treatment comprises a three-step programme:

➣ Learning relaxation skills, to be able to deal with the fear and anxiety the phobia presents. Typically, this might involve meditation and techniques for controlling one's breathing. These techniques allow the patient to control their fear rather than letting it build up to a potentially harmful level.

➤ Drawing-up a list of fears, rating their level of perceived threat, known as the 'anxiety hierarchy'. For instance seeing a dog on the telly might rate a 1 out of 10, whereas having the same mutt barking and slobbering all over you might merit a 10 and full phobic mode.

➤ Working through this list from the least to most threatening fear by a gradual exposure to the object of the phobia; maybe seeing a photo of, say the dog (to continue our example), before confronting it 'in the flesh', before handling it etc. the patient slowly overcomes their phobia, while the previously mentioned relaxation techniques (or 'coping strategies') give them the defence to be able to pursue this course of therapy.

Hypnotherapy

Now here's a therapy of which I have direct experience ... but we'll come to that later. In hypnotherapy, the therapist puts the phobia sufferer into a trance and makes suggestions that somehow register in the subconscious and affect the sufferer's subsequent attitudes and actions.

It's interesting to see the kinds of phobia that hypnotherapy is most often used to address. In the world of big business, and especially in the States, the fear of flying and the fear of public speaking are considered such an impediment to success in business that therapists can easily demand in excess of $1,000 a day for intensive one-on-one sessions (and if you work for a big corporation at a sufficiently high level, your employer will pick up the tab) and I'm sure the top rates are far higher. Outside the corporate environment, the most common reason to consult a therapist has to do with health matters. The desire to lose weight or quit smoking probably sends more people to hypnotherapists than any other motive.

In a recent TV series investigating alternative therapies, the presenter, Professor Kathy Sykes, watched a hypnotherapist work with members of the police who wanted to stop smoking. The therapist asked one subject, 'What's the worst thing that can happen if you smoke?' Then the policeman was made to repeat that he *would* get cancer, he *would* die, and he *would* leave his wife and children behind. This was worst-case scenario writ large: no "might" about it. Perhaps these extreme scare-tactics were geared to these tough northern cops; in any case, the subject repeated 'I don't smoke' several times and was brought round after an hour. Guess what? He seemed to have lost his craving for cigarettes.

If that wasn't heavy-handed enough, the therapist's treatment of the next patient – a woman whose fondness for chocolate had, not to put too fine a point on it, piled on the pounds – removed all doubt. The woman was hypnotised to believe (or more accurately *want* to believe) that her beloved chocolate had the smell, taste and texture of something she hated: corned beef. On being brought round, she was offered some chocolate, which duly made her gag.

Both of these demonstrations smacked of stage hypnotism. Both seemed more extreme than was warranted. Did the cop need to think he'd die if he carried on smoking? Did the woman have to be told that chocolate would make her sick? It seemed as though the therapist had neutralised two compulsions at the expense of turning them into phobias. Not craving chocolate is one thing, but feeling anxious about it is a dubious kind of remedy. Was it necessary to condition these people to hate what they used to love? Why not try to achieve a more impartial state of mind?

As Derren Brown says, 'if you have a fear of dogs, you don't want to replace it with an equally compulsive love of them; you want the presence of mind still to spot the occasional vicious one and leave it alone.' And perhaps the ability to treat yourself to the odd Mars bar without wanting to retch or feeling compelled to eat a box-load. For the record, the cop and the choco-holic both lasted several weeks after their single hypnotherapy session before succumbing to their respective addictions. Clearly, the threats of cancer and corned beef weren't sufficient deterrents, though they did stop these two people enjoying their lapses. Does that really qualify as a success story?

Some scientists question whether a hypnotic state even exists. Professor Irving Kirsch of the University of Hull believes that those who respond positively to sug-gestion will do so just as well outside a trance as within it. It appears some people are just more sus-ceptible to suggestion than others and we can leave it there, while Professor Amir Raz sees the term "trance" as woolly and vague and rejects "hypnosis," prefer-ring to describe his work as 'attentional manipulation.'

At the end of the TV documentary came a nod to the sensationalist side of hypnotherapy as we saw a woman called Mandy undergo a 90-minute dental procedure to extract two teeth with nothing more in the way of anaesthesia than the soothing voice of her dentist-cum-hypnotherapist. Mandy's pulse stayed steady throughout her ordeal, and she claimed to have suffered no pain. The presenter, film crew and viewing public, on the other hand, went into phobic freak-mode. Truly gruesome viewing, the programme did no favours for hypnotherapy.

Medication

As I have no knowledge of medicine whatsoever, it would be utterly irresponsible of me to write about or recommend anything. I would advise readers to turn to Richard Stern, whose *Mastering Phobias* includes a chapter on the role of medication. Anyone so adversely affected by a phobia that they are considering medication should see their doctor in any case. So should anyone already taking medication who thinks they might want to make changes to their personal regime.

Episode 2:
Tackling the library

Knowing about my phobias, my mate Ian introduced me to a friend of his called Ej who was training to be a hypnotherapist. We met and talked about our interests and what we'd hope to gain from our relationship. Having established a good rapport, we decided to set aside a day a week for the next few months to work on my phobia together.

Ej asked me to think about what affected me most. He wanted to see my phobia in action, and asked me to choose a location where I would feel in complete control of what happened. He promised me that he would never force me to do anything I was unsure of and reassured me that this wasn't about facing my demons; it was about easing off my overprotective subconscious mind.

Choosing a location wasn't easy. My phobia was rather specific: I was scared not of heights in general, but of level surfaces where you'd suddenly glimpse a drop below (less acrophobia, perhaps, than bathophobia, the fear of falling into depths.) The platform at Brighton station and Brighton Pier might have qualified – both are built from old timbers with gaps you can see between – but I rejected both these options as too flat: I needed somewhere with gradations in height.

So I went to the library. Brighton is justifiably proud of its new Jubilee Library, but this big open-plan building of glass and steel with open flights of stairs and see-through barriers represented my undoing. I couldn't even climb the stairs and was reduced to taking the lift, full of regret and self-loathing (I was the only person in it).

I'd found my nemesis.

Two weeks later, Ej and I stood at the entrance to the library. Armed with a camcorder, Ej was going to document my attempted ascent of the west face. When we asked for permission to film, a lovely lady in the book-shop told me she had once escorted a visitor to the second floor by lift as she too was scared of heights and unable to use the stairs. Her compassion and helpfulness impressed me. Looking up the stairs, I started to feel not scared, but a little silly. I was attracting attention, and that, coupled with the camera, made me feel as though I was taking part in some kind of melodrama.

I shouldn't have worried; as it turned out, my perform-ance was entirely natural. From the first step I felt that my world had been torn out from beneath me. I couldn't imagine for a moment that what I was doing was safe. I felt sick and light-headed as the ground and the people below receded with every step. My legs abandoned any pretence of strength or reliability. Walking in the air might be fun for the cartoon snowman, but this was not liberation, it was terror. Reaching the first landing brought some relief. I could slightly release my two-handed grip on the banister and breathe a little easier. But I still had another floor to climb.

The next phase of the ascent was worse. My fear increased as I got higher. I felt my legs give way and thought I would fall. Suddenly I was concerned for the safety of the people in the library below. I might kill someone.

At the time, all these thoughts seemed entirely rational. It didn't occur to me for a moment that they were in any way abnormal. I learnt a valuable lesson about phobias: everyone's fear is utterly real to them, however unfounded or bizarre it might seem to anyone else.

Ej filmed my journey and hesitant commentary. Not once did I worry about what he might be thinking or care about how ridiculous I looked. Ego and vanity vanished. I was simply too scared.

I remembered having heard that some travellers are said to mistrust people who live or work above ground level. They call them sky-dwellers. Right now I could understand their qualms.

Strangely enough, though, going down again was much easier. Grab a handrail, close your eyes, take small steps and let gravity do the rest.

Sitting in the pub afterwards, Ej gave me a list of questions. I thought he would ask how I was feeling after my ordeal, but the questions seemed completely random. What colour is your front door? What sort of car do you think I might drive?

Ej explained that he was looking at my eyes when I answered to see which of the six parts of the brain I was using. (If you think about the colour of your front door, you're likely to look up and to the left, for instance.) From my eye movements Ej could gauge whether I was more responsive to visual, audio or other stimuli and then devise a course of hypnotherapy tailored to my specific make-up. To this, he would add breathing exercises, anchoring (whatever that might be) and possibly some work on acupressure points.

After the therapy, we would re-test my reaction to the library. We had two months; Ej would have preferred three.

Agoraphobia and social phobias

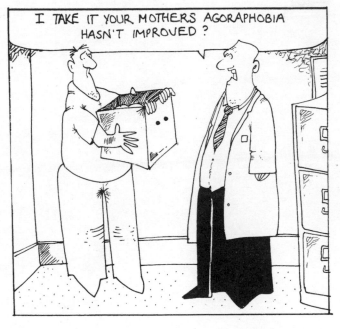

Throughout the rest of this book I've used the standard psychiatric categorisations as laid down in *The ICD-10 Classification of Mental and Behavioural Disorders* (1992), published by the World Health Organisation, as a way of structuring my thematic lists of phobias. However, this approach takes us only so far. As the number of phobias increases, more and more seem to elude easy classification and have to be placed under the catch-all heading 'other.' So I've augmented the official categories with subdivisions of my own invention such as 'the body.'

Agoraphobia

This is defined as an irrational anxiety about being in places from which escape might be difficult or embarrassing. It is often but not always accompanied by anxiety attacks. This is one of the commonest types of phobia, accounting for three-fifths of all phobias. The majority of sufferers – at least two-thirds – are women, usually between the ages of 15 and 35.

The following phobias fall into this category:

Being bound (or tied up)	Merinthophobia
Being buried alive (and cemeteries)	Taphephobia Taphophobia
Being smothered	Pnigerophobia
Cemeteries	Coimetrophobia
Churches	Ecclesiophobia
Confined and cramped spaces	Claustrophobia
Crowds	Agoraphobia Demophobia Enochlophobia Ochlophobia
Going to bed	Clinophobia
Going to school	Didaskaleinophobia Scolionophobia
Hospitals	Nosocomephobia
Houses (and being in them)	Domatophobia Ecophobia Eicophobia Oikophobia
Returning home	Nostophobia
Rooms (and being in them)	Koinoniphobia
Space	Spacephobia
Theatres	Theatrophobia

Claustrophobia and Taphephobia

The fear of being buried alive is common to most cultures and a mainstay of our horror tradition, specifically the Gothic.

Its pre-eminence as a horror motif can be shown by the fact Quentin Tarantino has used it twice in recent work. In *Kill Bill Vol. II* (2004), 'The Bride' (Uma Thurman) undergoes this terrifying ordeal, which Tarantino must have thought successful as he recycled it the following year for the two-part, season 5 finale of *CSI*, amusingly titled '*Grave Danger.*'

There is the literal fear, the immanent suffocating slow-death, best illustrated in Edgar Allen Poe's nerve-shredding *Premature Burial* and *The Fall of the House of Usher*, and the symbolic, representative of disturbed mental-states and a feeling of powerlessness at the external circumstances of life (similar to that which drowning also symbolises.) Pre psychiatry, Poe seemed to draw these strands together and in *Premature Burial* presents a man so obsessed by being buried alive, that the precautions he takes cease to satisfy and so becomes trapped within his own phobia. Although the story has a 'happy' ending, Poe/The Narrator survives his ordeal with a new sense of the joy of living; the irony of the title wasn't lost on Poe, the *Premature Burial* of the title refers as much to the helplessness of the phobic condition. In as much as a man can die many times before his death, so can he be 'buried-alive' many times as well.

Social phobias

Someone with a social phobia suffers irrational anxiety when exposed to certain types of social situation or performance, and may seek to avoid them. Although women are supposedly more phobic than men, one study found that over three-quarters of social phobia sufferers were men.

Here are some social phobias:

Accidents	Dystychiphobia
Being alone	Autophobia Monophobia
Being forgotten (or ignored or forgetting)	Athazagoraphobia
Being hypnotised (and sleep)	Hypnophobia
Being oneself (and loneliness)	Eremophobia
Being ridiculed	Catagelophobia Katagelophobia
Being severely punished, beaten or criticised	Rhabdophobia
Being single	Anuptaphobia
Being stared at	Ophiophobia Ophthalmophobia Scopophobia Scoptophobia
Being thought of negatively	Socialphobia
Being touched	Aphenphosmphobia Chiraptophobia Haphephobia Haptephobia
Blushing (and red things)	Ereuthophobia Ereuthrophobia Erythrophobia Erytophobia Eyrythrophobia

Body odour	Autodysomophobia Bromidrophobia Bromidrosiphobia Osphresiophobia
Challenges to or deviation from official doctrine	Hereiophobia Heresyphobia
Childbirth	Lockiophobia Maieusiophobia Parturiphobia Tocophobia
Chopsticks (and using them)	Consecotaleophobia
Constipation	Coprastasophobia
Cooking	Mageirocophobia
Dancing	Chorophobia
Death (and dead things and dying)	Necrophobia Thanatophobia Thantophobia
Defecation	Rhypophobia
Dependence on others	Soteriophobia
Dining (and dinner conversations)	Deipnophobia
Drinking	Dipsophobia
Expressing opinions (and receiving praise)	Doxophobia
Failure (and defeat)	Atychiphobia Kakorraphiaphobia Kakorrhaphiophobia

Fainting (and weakness)	Asthenophobia
Falling in love (and being in love)	Philophobia
Fatigue	Kopophobia
Firearms	Hoplophobia
Flogging	Mastigophobia
Food (and eating)	Cibophobia Sitiophobia Sitophobia
Foreign languages	Xenoglossophobia
Gaining weight	Obesophobia Pocrescophobia
Going bald	Phalacrophobia
Hearing certain words or names	Onomatophobia
Hearing good news	Euphobia
Hearing one's own voice on the telephone	Phonophobia Telephonophobla
Kissing	Philemaphobia Philematophobia
Laughter	Geliophobia
Lawsuits	Liticaphobia
Learning	Sophophobia
Long waits	Macrophobia
Losing an erection	Medomalacuphobia
Love play (and games)	Malaxophobia Sarmassophobia

Making decisions	Decidophobia
Marriage	Gametophobia Gamophobia
Meat	Carnophobia
Names	Nomatophobia
Neglecting duty (or responsibility)	Paralipophobia
Nudity	Gymnophobia Nudophobia
Opinions	Allodoxaphobia
Peanut butter being stuck to the roof of one's mouth	Arachibutyrophobia
Poverty	Peniaphobia
Preferring fearful situations	Counterphobia
Prescribing medication (suffered by doctors)	Opiophobia
Punishment	Mastigophobia Poinephobia
Rape	Virginitiphobia
Religious ceremonies	Teleophobia
Responsibility	Hypegiaphobia Hypengyophobia
Ridicule	Katagelophobia
Ruin	Atephobia
Sermons	Homilophobia
Sex	Genophobia

Sexual abuse	Agraphobia Contreltophobia
Sexual intercourse	Coitophobia
Sexual love	Erotophobia
Sexual perversion	Paraphobia
Sin (and sinning)	Enissophoia Enosiophobia Hamartophobia Harmatiophobia Peccatophobia
Singing	Canophobia
Sleep	Somniphobia
Soiling	Rypophobia
Solitude	Eremitophobia Eremophobia Isolophobia Monophobia
Speaking aloud (and noise)	Phonophobia
Speaking aloud (and stuttering)	Glossophobia Halophobia Laliophobia Lalophobia
Stealing	Cleptophobia Kleptophobia
Taking tests	Testophobia
Undressing in front of someone	Dishabiliophobia

Working on computers (and computers)	Cyberphobia Logizomechanophobia
Working with chemicals (and chemicals)	Chemophobia
Writing (and handwriting)	Graphophobia
Writing in public	Scriptophobia

Food and phobias

'Food, glorious food,' as a fictitious pre-pubescent Victorian orphan once warbled. And indeed food is glorious; though our taste in food is a complicated business that involves political, religious, sociological and cultural factors as well as the relatively straightforward matters of flavour, texture and aroma. Eating and sex are among the few biological imperatives that unite us, and yet both are fraught with confusion and indeed subject to multiple phobias.

I pride myself on having a rather bizarre food phobia: I'm scared of food with faces. A fast-food joint in my hometown of Brighton has a logo that terrifies me: a big burger with eyes on the top of its bun. On Hove seafront I see a van selling hog roasts decorated with a pig wearing a chef's apron and giving a cheeky wink and a cheery thumbs-up. My phobia is a curious blend of the aesthetic (anthropomorphising a burger is just ludicrous) and the moral (the implication that pigs might *want* you to eat them inflames my vegetarian sensibilities). But I have no objection to Jammy Dodgers or any other biscuits with faces – that would be just silly.

Meat

If you think about meat and where it comes from, it's hardly surprising that some people have a phobia about eating it. As someone once pointed out: 'the average person ... will respond positively to "tender juicy filet mignon" on the menu; but not to "a piece off of a dead castrated bull."'

Some people abstain from eating meat but don't mind fish, arguing that it's not as cruel because fish don't feel pain (which is dubious) or simply justifying their decision on the basis that fish is good for you (true, but still hard on the fish). We all determine our own comfort zone. What we want to eat, we can usually find a way to justify. Horse and Guinea Pig may not be on the menu in Britain but they are in France and Peru respectively, where as *Cuy*, (pronounced coo-ee) roast and utterly whole Guinea Pig is consumed to the tune of 65 million little furry-meals annually. It supposedly contains more protein and less fat than more commonly eaten meats and for once doesn't supposedly taste like chicken.

... It tastes like rat (to those who know these things).

Also in notoriously squeamish and conservative Britain, eel's not uncommon (which many find utterly unpalatable) and squirrel is apparently gaining in popularity.

(I'm so glad I don't eat such things!)

Just as some people can't stand eating meat, there are those who eat nothing else. Consider Nat Holland, who for most of her nineteen short years has lived solely on sausages so burnt that you'd need DNA evidence to identify them. This isn't meat; it's more like coal. Poor Nat says that trying any other food makes her gag, so she stays with what she knows and trusts. Apparently her parents indulged her eccentric taste when she was a child, as she'd suffered bronchial pneumonia and they wanted her to be happy.

Thanks to this exclusive diet of minced pigs' tails, noses and ears, Nat's salt intake was ten times the recommended limit, while her soaring cholesterol levels put her at risk of high blood pressure and heart disease. But her story has a happy ending. She has been helped to overcome her cibophobia by being taught to put small pieces of new foods in her mouth, get familiar with the new tastes and slowly begin to chew and swallow small pieces. Having learnt how to eat again from scratch, she now tackles a more varied diet embracing pasta, pizza, cheese and eggs. Hmm – no fresh fruit or veg there, but lots of fat. Maybe eating coal isn't so bad after all.

Fruit and vegetables

One of my college friends, who seems a sensible sort of chap, wouldn't eat fresh fruit or vegetables because he was scared of what he might find under the skin when he bit into it. Would a pear be as raw as a potato or liquefied mush? The mere thought unnerved him, so he acted like any phobic person and avoided all possible encounters with the objects of his fears, regardless of the implications for his health.

Chris Hawkins used to suffer from the same phobia. By the time he started school, he'd stopped eating fruit and vegetables; by the time he'd sought treatment, his phobia was so bad he couldn't go anywhere near a greengrocer or the fresh produce aisle at a supermarket. His wife had to store fruit and veg separately and out of sight, and keep a special set of knives for preparing them. When he was eating out, no only did he have to go to great lengths to find things he could eat, but he also had to take pains not to look at what other people were eating around him.

Apparently tomatoes had the worst effect: just seeing or smelling them made him feel physically sick. In fact, aversion to tomatoes seems to be the most common of all the specific food phobias I've encountered.

When Chris, who was a DJ, referred to his phobia on air, he was inundated with calls and messages of support. He eventually undertook a cure in the form of a four-week course that included paragliding, treading grapes and eating in the dark. The results were impressive: he replaced his beloved coffee with fruit smoothies and managed to prepare a vegetable curry.

Episode 3:
Two sessions with Ej

It's a week after my attempted assault on the library, and the start of my first session with Ej. We begin with a visualisation exercise. I shut my eyes, slow down my breathing and try to relax. My body feels both looser and heavier. I have to think of someone I respect and admire and imagine meeting him or her at a party. The idea is to try to take on the self-confidence that my chosen role model exudes.

I find myself in a passive receptive state. One part of me enjoys it, another is wary of how vulnerable I am.

We've been working for only about twenty-five minutes when I smile, maybe even laugh, at the thought of the person I have in mind being scared of heights. This is easy – I'm already cured!

Not so fast. Ej explains that he is trying to help me build a memory in my body so that it can understand what it feels like to be without fear. The idea is that I should be able to call up this memory whenever I am in a situation that would normally trigger my phobia.

The second part of the treatment involves various hypnotherapeutic techniques. They seem very powerful. For someone with poor visualisation abilities, I do a good job of stumbling and falling in my own front room. I feel I am actually back in the library at that point and it is quite unsettling.

Six days later

Ej's treatment stirred up strange spirits in me. I can remember this happening only once before, after psychic healing. Troubling images disturbed my sleep: not the terror of nightmares, but a litany of all the rotten things I'd ever done. It felt as though my subconscious was throwing up. But would it have any purgative effect?

One curious consequence is that I suddenly feel I have an inkling of what might have triggered my phobia. I've always been a big fan of the classic prison-life TV sitcom Porridge, *which I've watched since I was a kid. In the opening sequence, old lag Fletcher, played by*

Ronnie Barker, gravely proclaims his own sentence: 'Norman Stanley Fletcher, you have pleaded guilty to the charges brought by this court and it is now my duty to pass sentence ... You will go to prison for five years.' The prisoner is led clanking up wrought-iron steps to his cell, whereupon we hear the sound of the jailer's key in the lock.

Until then, I'd regarded Porridge *as comfort viewing. I'd never been aware of the open stairs and the way they end in Fletch's loss of freedom. I'd seen this opening sequence a thousand times and never linked it to my phobia until now. It struck me too that having Fletch double as his own judge revealed the man's self-loathing and self-condemnation. So was that what my phobia was all about?*

The second session

Ej starts me off with a repeat of the previous week's visualisation exercise. The next step is anchoring: imagining a safe, happy place that you can always return to when you need to feel calm. Once I would have chosen a beach in Hawaii that I'd visited some years earlier. Now my mind conjures up a picture of domestic bliss: nice flat, girlfriend, cat ... I can even feel the heat from the oven. Alas, bliss had proved short-lived and Ej brings me back from this idyll on the verge of tears. Clearly it's safer to stick with Honolulu.

We end with some hypnotherapy proper. I drift for over half an hour, not knowing if I am awake or asleep, but still hearing Ej's soporific voice.

Well, something's going on. I feel great. *Now all I have to do is walk up two flights of stairs. Then we'll see how confident I really am.*

Animals, people, dummies and the like

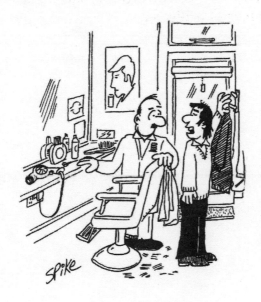

'CUT BOTH SHORT,
HAIR AND THE CONVERSATION!'

cartoonstock.com

The rest of the phobias I look at in this book qualify as 'specific phobias': 'those characterised by persistent and irrational fear in the presence of some specific stimulus which often prompts the sufferer to withdraw in order to avoid it.'

Types of specific phobia include:

➤ **Animals** – the subject of this chapter. I've also added two sub-types, 'People' and 'Dummies and the like.' I look at the remaining specific phobias in later chapters:

➤ **Features of the natural environment** such as storms, heights or water.

➤ **Fears of blood, injection or injury** cued by witnessing some invasive medical procedure.

➤ **Particular situations** such as public transport, tunnels, bridges, lifts, flying, driving or enclosed spaces.

➤ **Other types** including choking, vomiting or contracting an illness.

I've also taken the liberty of adding the following categories to cover phobias that don't seem to fit neatly within the official classification:

➤ **The arts and sciences**
➤ **The body**
➤ **The emotional and philosophical**
➤ **Religion and superstition.**

And even then I had to give up and label a few as "Miscellaneous" – sorry.

Animals

I'm afraid it's official; some things are just scarier than others.

Martin Seligman's showed how more people had adverse reactions to picture of snakes than flowers and established the hypothesis that 'certain objects might have a genetic predisposition to being associated with fear.'

The biology of this is that on being confronted with the object (or representation of the object) of our fears, an area of our brain, called the amygdala, produces hormones which puts our bodies into an 'alert state', ready for 'fight-or-flight.' This is seen as 'an unnatural or illogical functioning of the brain.'

Amphibians	Batrachophobia
Animals	Zoophobia
Ants	Myrmecophobia
Bacteria	Bacteriophobia
Bees	Apiphobia Melissophobia
Birds	Ornithophobia
Bones, fur and skins	Doraphobia
Bulls	Taurophobia
Cats	Ailurophobia Elurophobia Felinophobia Galeophobia Gatophobia
Chickens	Alektorophobia
Dogs	Canophobia Cynophobia
Feathers (and being tickled by them)	Pteronophobia
Fish	Icthyophobia
Frogs	Ranidaphobia
Great mole rat	Zemmiphobia
Horses	Equinophobia Hippophobia
Insects	Entomophobia Insectophobia

Insects (and itching caused by them)	Acarophobia
Lice	Pediculophobia Phthiriophobia
Meat	Carnophobia
Mice	Muriphobia Musophobia Suriphobia
Microbes	Bacilliophobia Bacillophobia Microbiophobia
Moths	Mottephobia
Otters	Lutraphobia
Parasites	Parasitophobia
Reptiles	Batrachophobia Herpetophobia
Sharks	Selachophobia
Shellfish	Ostraconophobia
Snakes	Ophidiophobia Ophiophobia Snakephobia
Spiders	Arachnaphobia Arachnephobia Arachnophobia
Stings	Cnidophobia
Tapeworms	Taeniophobia Teniophobia
Termites	Isopterophobia

Toads	Bufonophobia
Wasps	Spheksophobia
Wild animals	Agrizoophobia
Worms	Helminthophobia Scoleciphobia

No lions, tigers, hippos, rhinos or elephants? Or are they all covered under 'Wild animals'? Come to think of it, these are all dangerous animals and fearing or running away from them wouldn't constitute a phobia; you'd be mad *not* to be scared of them. If you look at the animals in the list of phobias, none of them poses much threat to us. Well, hardly any (sharks, snakes, spiders, and what about wasps? Nobody likes them). Domestic animals may seem a strange thing to be afraid of, but many of us have had unpleasant encounters with dogs and even horses.

Now I think about it, otters are fairly creepy. Maybe it's their human-looking paws?

And what about my next subject – the great mole rat?

Zemmiphobia

For anyone unfamiliar with this creature, let me borrow a definition from urbandictionary.com:

> "An obscure and mysterious mole rat that takes presence in the rituals and practices of many underground cults esp. in the New Mexico area. In the Blood Eyes cult the great mole rat is seen as a symbol of shame."

Zemmiphobia regularly makes the top 10 lists of the weirdest phobias. There's just one tiny problem: the great mole rat doesn't seem to exist. I found more than 714 pages in English on the internet that make some mention of it, but every one serves merely to alert us to the fact that some people are scared of them. When I searched for the great mole rat without the words 'fear of' I was left with a single solitary reference: a domain name called www.greatmolerat.com, which can be yours for the paltry sum of US$650. Tempting!

Admittedly, there is a naked mole rat, described by an expert in the following glowing terms: 'Endowed with pinkish-grey, wrinkly skin, scant hair, and long buck teeth, naked mole-rats ... aren't likely to win any beauty contests. Some might refer to them as down-right ugly, resembling an overcooked hotdog with teeth.' As these three-inch long critters spend virtually their entire lives deep in African soil, they're unlikely to have many devotees in New Mexico, and they hardly qualify as great. Indeed, they pull off the difficult stunt of offending both creationists and Darwinists at the same time, as well as single-handedly refuting the concept of intelligent design. It's hard to tell if they evolved underground or were driven there by a lynch mob of better-looking rodents.

So rely on the Internet at your peril. As many people have noted, once something's out there in cyberspace it gets quoted, re-quoted, elaborated and commented on until it acquires a life of its own. I reckon someone made up the great mole rat invention for a laugh and submitted it to phobialist.com. Once it appeared there, legions of phobia fans picked it up and so zemmiphobia and its definition have been reposted on hundreds of other sites. That's my theory; prove me wrong if you can.

People

Amputees	Apotemnophobia
Bad men (and burglars)	Scelerophobia
Bald people	Peladophobia
Beautiful women	Caligynephobia Venustraphobia
Beggars (and tramps)	Hobophobia
Black people (and culture)	Melanophobia Negrophobia
Bogeymen	Bogyphobia
Bolsheviks	Bolshephobia
Children (and dolls)	Paedophobia Pedophobia
Chinese people (and culture)	Sinophobia
Clowns	Coulrophobia
Deformed (children and monsters)	Teratophobia
Dentists (and going to the dentist)	Dentophobia
Doctors (and going to the doctor)	Iatrophobia
Dutch people (and culture)	Dutchnophobia
English people (and culture)	Anglophobia

Europeans (and European culture)	Europhobia
Foreigners	Xenophobia
French people (and culture)	Francophobia Galiophobia Gallophobia
Germans (and German culture)	Germanophobia Teutophobia
Homosexuals	Homophobia
Japanese people (and culture)	Japanophobia
Jewish people (and culture)	Judeophobia
Men	Androphobia Anthropophobia Arrhenphobia Hominophobia
Moslems (and Islamic culture)	Islamaphobia
Old people (and growing old)	Gerontophobia
Opposite sex	Heterophobia Sexophobia

Some years ago, the compassionate and enlightened psychologists of the University of Arkansas decided that 'Homophobia is not an actual phobia because it's caused by disgust, not fear or anxiety.' So now you know. If I've got any gay readers, I suggest you get onto those southern banjo-heads and show them what real disgust is.

Parents-in-law	Soceraphobia
People and society	Anthropophobia Sociophobia
Politicians	Politicophobia
Popes	Papaphobia
Priests (and holy things)	Hierophobia
Relatives	Syngenesophobia
Robbers (and being robbed)	Harpaxophobia
Russians (and Russian culture)	Russophobia
Saints (and holy relics)	Hagiophobia
Satan	Satanophobia
Stepfather	Vitricophobia
Stepmother	Novercaphobia Pentheraphobia
Teenagers	Ephebiphobia
Tyrants	Tyrannophobia
Virgins (and young girls)	Parthenophobia
Walloons	Walloonphobia
Witches (and witchcraft)	Wiccaphobia
Women	Gynephobia Gynophobia

Most wanted

There seem to be a few striking omissions from this list. What, no nuns? And how about families?

It's time we had names for phobias of:

Parents
Partners of any hue (especially exes – how about bunniboilaphobia?)
Grandparents and grandchildren
Teachers (and let's have a separate one for games teachers – they know they deserve it).

In fact, the list of 'People' phobias is revealing: traditional fears of the deformed and the 'other', coupled with fears of historically antagonistic European powers, World War II combatants, Cold War enemies and the new super-powers. Curiously, the Italians, Spanish and Portuguese don't seem to annoy anyone enough to warrant their own phobia names even in a list with such an Anglocentric bias. Perhaps we should be surprised there aren't more peoples and races singled out for fear and aversion.

The Russians enjoy the dubious distinction of getting a second look-in with the anachronistic fear of Bolsheviks, and we can only wonder at what Walloons

(French-speaking Belgians) have done to inspire fear, unless you count Jacques Brel. Yet there's no name for the phobia of America and Americans. Is that because no one's scared of them? Nor is there a fear of presidents, unless it's covered by tyrannophobia.

Oh, and mime artistes really do deserve to be up there with the clowns.

Peladophobia

Why do people fear and hate the bald? I should confess a personal interest here, having been bald for over a decade.

Going bald can be perceived as passive, weak, resigned. Choosing to go bald, on the other hand, can be empowering. Both the artist Pablo Picasso and the infamous occultist Aleister Crowley started losing their hair early in life. After trying out unconvincing comb-overs and hats, each of them eventually bit the bullet and went for the full chop, so creating two of the twentieth century's most iconic images of bald geniuses with mad hypnotic eyes. Without hair to conceal or accentuate, the face's features are laid bare.

Making another person bald can be seen as a sign of oppression: something done by the state to prisoners or the condemned. Forcibly shaving off someone's hair dehumanises them and makes them easier to despise and ignore. Shaving your own head, on the other hand, can be seen as a sign of toughness and aggression. Soldiers, boxers and martial arts enthusiasts often have shaven heads.

Baldness can sometimes be associated with taking a vow. Whether they are Christian, Buddhist or Hindu, monks often shave their heads. It marks them out as different, unconcerned with earthly vanity. Some Zen monks even shave off their eyebrows.

(On the other hand, Rastafarians and Sikhs never cut their hair, so there's a limit to how far you can take the religious connection.)

Of course, balding is a sign of ageing and mortality. It can be caused by illness and is a distressing side effect of some cancer treatments. Balding is also associated with madness. What was the most shocking aspect of Britney Spears' recent troubles? Shaving her head, which was widely seen as proof of a breakdown. Perhaps she was simply trying to leave her pop image behind, and believed that being bald would make her ugly.

Some actors have found baldness isn't exactly a career asset. When Samuel L. Jackson became an overnight star in 1994, it was partly because of a wig. His Oscar-nominated role as Jules in *Pulp Fiction* might never have had the impact it did without a little follicular assistance. An early publicity still of the film cast shows him with a bald patch and widow's peak. By the time Quentin Tarantino shot the film, Jackson had been kitted out with a killer Afro as befitted the coolest of hit men. Jules needed hair to make him funkier, hipper, and more charismatic.

And take Sean Connery. Although he had Bond's looks, physique and magnetism, he didn't have 007's hair and had to wear a succession of wigs. As time went on, he resorted to them less and less and started to take pride in his age. Much the same thing happened with Bruce Willis too. (Villains are another matter. Baldness can be a positive boon: consider Blofeld, best immortalised by Donald Pleasence in *You Only Live Twice*, bald and disfigured – two phobias for the price of one.)

Comics of the Marvel ilk have long been solid repositories of peladophobia. Superheroes (or rather their alter-egos) have full heads of hair (Clark Kent, Peter Parker, Reed Richards) while their various enemies (Lex Luthor, the Kingpin, the Leader, the Puppet Master) are slapheads to a man. What conclusion can we draw from this? That bald men are intelligent but driven mad or megalomaniac by bitterness? (At this point honesty obliges me to concede that there are in fact two bald superheroes: the Silver Surfer, who is an alien, and Charles Xavier, Professor X, stunning intellect and leader of the X-Men.)

Baldness may be ugly to some, but don't be scared of us. To be bald is to embrace contradictions. One of the most heart-warming images in recent years was the sight of the England football team taking off for the Euro 2000 tournament. To a man, they all had fresh skinhead cuts and flew the cross of St George. What had once been the symbol of an odious exclusivity was now a badge of honour for all to celebrate. They still played like crap though.

Coulrophobia

The worst reaction I've ever witnessed to any phobia was on an American chat show called *Maury*. Various guests were trundled out to be confronted with their worst fears. Cue the usual suspects: spiders, wigs and of course clowns. One of the studio guests was your archetypal American redneck. Overweight, bearded and baseball-capped, he could have been a biker, a trucker or just a guy you go fishing with. He looked comfortable enough until the clown walked onto the set. Then he went wild, screamed and cried, jumped from his seat, ran off the stage and leapt with admirable aplomb over a crash barrier. He was last seen stumbling from the studio an emotional wreck. He never looked back. It was as good an example of the flight reflex as you'll ever see.

Clowns seem genuinely bewildered by the antagonism they provoke, and understandably get a little defensive. They can also be astonishingly arrogant, if these thoughts on the clown's role are any guide: 'A clown can go anywhere and you can be part of any situation ... the clown is like ... a thermometer testing the temperature of how comfortable people are with themselves' or, as one American clown put it, 'There are no rules ... I'm a clown, there is no wrong.'

As with many phobias, coulrophobia may be rooted in the sufferer's past. If clowns are funny in theory (and it's a big 'if'), then the childhood reality can often be very different. 'When I was eight, my mom took me to the circus ... all through the show this one clown kept looking at me. He even pointed once ... anyway I had to go to the bathroom ... I heard footsteps, HUGE footsteps on the floor ... that's when I saw the two big red feet. I screamed, I screamed loud.' Or consider the experience of this boy of six: 'a clown got right up in my face and I could see his beard stubble under his make-up. He smelled bad and his eyes were weird ... I guess I never got over it.'

Let's face it; some clowns are just plain evil. Consider two archetypal evil clowns from fact and fiction: John Wayne Gacy, sometime children's party performer in the guise of Pogo or Patches the clown and Chicago serial killer circa 1975 to 1978, and Pennywise the Clown from Stephen King's *It*.

Although Gacy never committed his crimes made-up as a clown ('motley and slap'), what had previously been seen as charitable and philanthropic perform-ances were now seen as proof of his foul and perverted ways, in an interpretation, which other pro-fessions of convicted serial killers seem to avoid. To my knowledge most people still have faith in their doctors despite Harold Shipman being Britain's most notori-ous and numerous killer.

The example of John Wayne Gacy goes to show our already-formed prejudices against the clown, merely waiting for validation.

I'd argued that many people's coulrophobia came either from reading *It* or seeing the unforgettable TV adaptation in the 80s, starring Tim Curry as the eponymous villain.

But the clown is only one of many forms this ancient and malevolent creature takes. The only difference between the clown and the spider/werewolf/abusive adult form *It* takes is that all the other manifestations have been seen previously by at least one of the terrorised children, most notably in their beloved B-movies. If I may be so bold as to quote myself; 'Only Pennywise has an independent existence, and the reader becomes complicit in a secret known by children yet forgotten by adults – that clowns are *inherently* scary.'

But my explanation for the wholly fictitious origins of the 'Killer Clown' wasn't satisfying to many. Some argued that the fear of clowns as abductors, paedophiles and murderers had entered urban mythology by the early 1980s and Stephen King was in fact reflecting this panic rather than creating it. A commentator called Theo Paijmans speculates that these moral panics are cyclical in nature and may represent modern updates of much older tales like that of the Pied Piper of Hamelin or rumours of child abduction by gypsies and travelling circuses, a view endorsed by Dave Dennis in a letter to *Fortean Times*: 'Surely the clown, as the most easily identifiable member of the circus troupe, is tainted with the mistrust that seems to be the lot of transients, becoming the focus for fears of having our children stolen and our sedentary way of life challenged.'

Like a perverted version of 'the chicken and the egg' conundrum we have to ask, 'which came first, the clown or the fear?'

Or maybe it's a whole lot simpler than that. You can't help noticing that clowns look different: 'the white face and rictus grin of the clown ... resemble an animated corpse.' Maybe it's all down to the make-up. Underneath the painted smile we search in vain for the clown's real emotional state. Slabbed-on slap 'renders the observer impotent in measuring facial expression as a precursor of action .... When we observe the "happy clown" performing some aggressive behaviour, it becomes too much to take, creating intense confusion and fear.' We don't even need to resort to cod psychology: 'clowns by nature are very scary things .... The size of the nose, the make-up, the lips, the hair, the smile ... to a kid, it is what a monster looks like.'

Perhaps we'd look more kindly on clowns if the humour they ply were more relevant; it's arguable that clown phobia increases with time as clowns become more anachronistic, like old-time music-hall acts. If we can't share the clown's sense of humour, what's left? Just the ludicrous and terrifying trappings of his profession.

If clowns are scary at the best of times, imagine the effect they must have in hospitals when they wander the paediatric wards to cheer up all the little patients (whoever came up with that therapeutic gem?). A recent poll conducted by the University of Sheffield of 250 children between the ages of 4 and 16 found that 'all of them disliked clowns as part of hospital décor, with even the oldest children finding them scary.' And a child psychologist found that very few children like clowns, believing that 'they don't look funny, they just look odd.'

Dummies and the like

Dolls	Pediophobia
Puppets	Pupaphobia
Ventriloquists' dummies (and the like)	Automatonophobia

It seems we often fear the things we make in our own image. The dread of statues, dolls, mannequins, scarecrows, action figures, marionettes, ventriloquists' dummies, robots, androids and indeed anything resembling humans is known as automatonophobia. From *Pygmalion* to *Pinocchio*, *Bladerunner* to *A.I.*, the story's the same: we create perfect companions who then become all too human, decide they don't need us any more and leave us behind physically, intellectually and emotionally.

Ever since *Frankenstein* (of which more shortly), automatonophobia has been a staple of the horror genre: vampires, zombies and mummies all play to this fear. At the height of the Cold War, dread of the enemy within took the phenomenon to new levels of paranoia with *Invasion of the Body Snatchers* (originally released in 1956, remade in 1978 and 2007) and *Village of the Damned* (1960, 1995) based on John Wyndham's 1957 sci-fi classic *The Midwich Cuckoos*. Does the host of remakes prove the perennial power of automatonophobia, or is it just that no one has original ideas any more?

Still, it's a haunting refrain: 'our children hate us. They want to kill us.'

Ventriloquism has also made numerous appearances on the silver screen, from the early *The Great Garbo*

(1929) through *Dead of Night* (1945) and *Devil Doll* (1964) to *Magic* (1978, but William Goldman's book was better). I suppose I have to mention the inexplicably popular *Child's Play* series of movies (1988 to the present), which holds the dubious distinction of tapping into more variants of automatonophobia than anything else on our list with the honourable exception of *Frankenstein*.

TV too has seen its share of dummies. Many a childhood has doubtless been blighted by Keith Harris and the egregious Orville (a fat hairy green duck, if you have managed to suppress the memories), while those who saw suave chat show host Michael Parkinson being savaged by Emu with a little assistance from Rod Hull won't need reminding that dummies can be vicious creatures.

US sitcom *Soap* featured a taciturn character called Chuck who let his little wooden friend voice his hostility and aggression. The idea that dummies are in some way licensed to say and do what their human operators can't is widespread: as one ventriloquist put it, 'Everything that I think I can't say, it comes through her and if she says it, it's OK. If I were to say it, it wouldn't be.'

The secret of good ventriloquism? According to the head of the British Association of Ventriloquists, it's *'Keep them living all the time.'* Chilling.

When you couple up automatonophobia with techno-phobia, things can get even darker. In his excellent book *Techgnosis*, Erik Davis argues that technological innovation, far from having a rationalising and demys-tifying effect on the human psyche, in fact widens the scope for dread by channelling people's deepest fears into new vehicles. He links the Victorians' obsession with spiritualism to the rise of the telegraph: as a new technology came into being, people responded by seeking out a kind of occult equivalent to it.

Undoubtedly the granddaddy of the whole science-fiction 'man or machine' tradition is Mary Shelley's *Frankenstein*, written in 1816 when experiments with electricity and the exploration of the human body through dissection were the order of the day. In con-versations with her husband, the poet Percy Bysshe Shelley, and their friend Lord Byron, Mary Shelley speculated that 'Perhaps a corpse would be reani-mated; galvanism had given token of such things: perhaps the component parts of a creature might be manufactured, brought together and endued with vital warmth.' Dr Frankenstein's wayward creation has seldom left our screens since, although Robert De Niro's portrayal of the monster in Kenneth Branagh's

Mary Shelley's Frankenstein (1994) could very nearly have marked its final throes. But thankfully the fascination has proved more robust. As the far superior original movie from 1931 rightfully declared, 'A monster science created, but could not destroy.'

(If Frankenstein's monster truly scares you, a cure is close at hand. Simply play the 'Putting on the Ritz' scene from Mel Brooks' *Young Frankenstein* (1974) as often as required until symptoms abate. Like Nazis, monsters have no defence against laughter.)

As Erik Davis correctly surmised, advances in technology have bred more complex fears concerning people's relationships with robots and robotics. Some of these fears surface in the multitude of robot-related TV series and films produced in recent years.

On TV, there's been the *Six Million Dollar Man* (1973–78) and *Bionic Woman* (1976–78), plus of course the Borg from *Star Trek: The Next Generation* (1987–94), and from this side of the pond those *Doctor Who* staples the Cybermen and the Autons, not to mention the more recent clockwork droids and weeping angels.

In film, take your pick from Bishop in *Alien* (1979), the replicants in *Bladerunner* (1982), *Terminator* (1984), *Robocop* (1987), *Artificial Intelligence: A.I.* (2001) and *I, Robot* (2004).

One question I'm compelled to ask is why cyborgs are made to look so attractive. After all, there is no need for them to have the faces and bodies of more perfect versions of ourselves unless they are being created as some sort of pleasure unit. I'm not alone in having been struck by this. Artificial intelligence expert David Levy predicts that by 2050 people will be having 'long-term sexual and emotional relationships with robots.' These newly improved sex dolls (which is what they come down to) will appeal mostly to 'men with low self-esteem, or men who want to objectify and control.' Now there's a surprise. As if pornography, prostitution and people trafficking weren't enough, now it looks as though the sex trade will be getting its hands on some of the most sophisticated technologies ever devised and using them for its own ends. So much for progress.

The cyborg as passive, sex-object is possibly best explored in *The Stepford Wives*, Ira Levin's 1972 novel, filmed in 1975, starring Katharine Ross and the Nicole Kidman remake from 2004.

The plot, (one of the staples of the entire horror genre), concerns 'townies', forced to relocate to a smaller, more rural, community.

(*You ain't from round these parts, are you boy?* As someone once actually said to me in Memphis.)

86

Joanna Eberhart, a sophisticated, New York photographer, not only finds the women of Stepford to be; 'fawning, submissive … (and) … impossibly beautiful', but also sees how friends become 'mindless', on taking up residence in the small town. In fact, the sinister reality is that the 'Wives' are not merely docile, but are actually 'gynoids', or perfectly life-like robots, created by the Stepford men-folk, a motley collection of scientists and engineers. The 'real' wives have simply been replaced.

Following Ms. Eberhart's uncovering of this murderous conspiracy, she fears for her life until the story ends with her 'assimilation' into the community as a perfect model of Stepford passivity and compatibility.

No happy endings here; Scientists with Robots 1, Human Beings 0.

Despite its modern themes *The Stepford Wives* is quaintly anachronistic, tapping-into older, Cold War scenarios like *Invasion of the Body-Snatchers* and *Village of the Damned* (*Midwich Cuckoos.*)

Previously-mentioned film and TV treatments of the book have followed various trajectories; 1) the women aren't killed and replaced, merely brain-washed and hypnotised, 2) the women are utterly brain-dead, vacuous and gorgeous, 3) in a 1996 TV movie the roles are reversed and it's the boys' turn to be turned into fantasy spouses and 4) the most recent remake (2004), even featured a gay clone (pun intended.)

Whatever the genders and orientations of the changing cast of characters, *The Stepford Wives* serves to remind us that when the technology exists to create and mould our ultimate sexual partners, we'll go ahead and do just that, gleefully amoralistically.

As human beings, we assume we have dominion over our robotic creations. We made them; we are free to destroy them. Over time, though, as many of these fictions suggest, the line between human and machine gets more and more blurred and we come to realise that what we took for a tool that would do our bidding has come to be our implacable enemy. Robots can enslave, assimilate or destroy us. As one character memorably warned from the depths of her secure psychiatric unit: 'they are coming and they are faster and stronger and they have been built to do one perfect thing ... to kill you .... They will kill everyone you love and everyone you hold close and there is nothing you can do about it .... They will find you because that's what they do ... they always do.'

Perhaps the 'point of singularity' – the moment when computers finally outsmart their human creators and render us all superfluous – isn't that far away.

According to one technology expert, it will take only a couple of decades for computers to match the power of the human brain. As silicon-based technology follows the law of accelerating returns, we can expect the next half-century to produce *32 times* more technical advances than the previous one (assuming there's any fuel around to power anything, that is).

So does fear of robots qualify as a phobia, or is it rather a perfectly rational response to a genuine threat? Only time will tell ...

Episode 4: Remember this feeling

On Sunday I go to the market near Brighton station as I've done many times over the past 25 years. But this time, I don't stumble when I glimpse the drop between the timbers on the dilapidated railway platform. I'm deep in conversation and don't even notice until I'm safely back on the main concourse. Does that mean I'm getting somewhere?

Let's hope so. What I most resent about my phobias is the time they waste. They are so unproductive. I wouldn't say working makes me happy, but inactivity is a kind of prison.

My next session. It's good to see Ej. His smile and optimism are infectious. I realise that someone I met only a couple of weeks ago knows me better than perhaps anyone else in the world does right now.

'This is how your body wants to feel. It loves this feeling, it remembers this feeling.'

Here we are at the start of the session doing my visualisation exercise. In my mind, my strong, charismatic role model stands before me. I try to adopt his posture and confident attitude.

'If in doubt, take the stance. Things will change.'

I'm meeting my role model at a party. Each session, I add further details. I can see what the guests are wearing, hear the music, and eavesdrop on conversations.

'For no apparent reason, you are feeling super-confident. Breathe in …'

Cough, splutter, gag. It's not the first time that's happened. The session seems to be going well and suddenly my body tries to sabotage it. It's as though the nasty little negative part of me wants attention and won't give up without a fight.

'Breathe in, breathe out. With each breath, feel the energy and confidence flowing through your body. Clear your mind. In a moment you're going somewhere I know you'll

want to be. Let your body remember what it's like. Once your body and your mind know that sensation I'll teach you ways of bringing it on. Here you are, you're outside Brixton Academy. You look up at the billboard and who's playing? It's the Ramones. Can you believe it?'

It was 1977 and I was a kid, soon to become part of the punk generation. I guess we can't choose the soundtrack to our formative years. Back then I was still listening to the Beatles and even ELO. But that was about to change.

'You've never been to a gig before; you can feel the energy, the buzz, the noise of the crowd. It's all so exciting and it's rubbing off on you.'

There's a roar of celebration and defiance. The stage goes dark; a revolving light picks out the giant eagle on the backdrop and the chanting starts.

'You know why you're here, but you've never experienced anything like this before. You can smell the excitement.'

Nervous energy tinged with anxiety surges through me. I can feel sweat on the back of my neck.

'This is what it feels like to be alive, this is how ecstatic you can feel, you never knew you could feel this good, you never knew you could feel this happy.'

Ej takes my feeling, doubles it, and trebles it.

'Every cell in your body loves this feeling and wants to be you at this gig. Remember it. You were there; you know what it felt like. Put it back into your memory. You can call on it whenever you want, go back to this gig whenever you want, remember this feeling.'

Thank you, Ej. Now I possess a positive memory so strong I can will myself into energy and confidence.

Stop press

My dad's just phoned to tell me that a new phobia has been named: nomophobia or the fear of being parted from one's mobile phone. It was only a matter of time. Apparently the best cure is to turn the damn thing off and get a life.

Nature, injury and situations

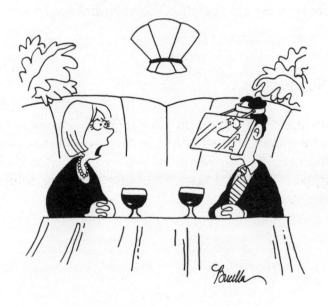

'I CAN ACCEPT THAT YOU'RE A GERMAPHOBE,
BUT I JUST CAN'T GET PAST THE SNEEZE GUARD.'

cartoonstock.com

Natural environment

Think of a natural phenomenon.

Do you find it beautiful?

Chances are, somewhere in the world, someone just like you, views it with utter horror ...

Alcohol	Methyphobia Potophobia
Asymmetrical things	Asymmetriphobia
Being cold (and cold things)	Cheimaphobia Cheimatophobia Frigophobia Psychrophobia
Clouds	Nephophobia
Colours	Chromatophobia Chromophobia Cromophobia
Comets	Cometophobia
Cosmic phenomena	Kosmikophobia
Crystals and glass	Crystallophobia
Dampness	Hygrophobia
Darkness	Achluophobia Achulophobia Lygophobia Myctophobia Nyctophobia Scotophobia
Dawn (and daylight)	Eosophobia
Daylight (and sunshine)	Phengophobia
Depths	Bathophobia
Dryness	Xerophobia
Dust	Amathophobia Koniphobia Koniophobia

Electricity	Electrophobia
Feeling dizzy when looking down	Illyngophobia
Fire	Arsonphobia Pyrophobia
Flashes	Seiaphobia Selaphobia
Floods	Antlophobia
Flowers	Anthophobia Anthrophobia
Fog	Homichlophobia Nebulaphobia
Forests (and wooden objects)	Hylophobia Xylophobia
Garlic	Alliumophobia
Gold	Aurophobia
Gravity	Barophobia
Heat	Thermophobia
Heights	Acrophobia Altophobia Hypsiphobia Hypsophobia
Ice (and frost)	Cryophobia Pagophobia
Jumping from high (or low) places	Catapedaphobia
Lakes	Limnophobia
Large things	Megalophobia

Leaves	Phyllophobia
Light	Photophobia
Liquids, dampness and moisture	Hygrophobia
Loud noises	Ligyrophobia
Metal	Metallophobia
Meteors	Meteorophobia
Moon	Selenophobia
Mushrooms	Mycophobia
Night	Noctiphobia Nyctophobia
Noise (and sound)	Acousticophobia
Northern lights	Auroraphobia
Open high spaces	Aeroacrophobia
Outer space	Spacephobia
Paper	Papyrophobia
Plants	Botanophobia
Precipices	Cremnophobia
Purple (and purple things)	Porphyrophobia
Rain (and being rained on)	Ombrophobia Pluviophobia
Rivers (and running water)	Potamophobia
Rust	Iophobia
Sea	Thalassophobia
Sea swell	Cymophobia

Shadows	Sciaphobia Sciophobia
Slime	Blennophobia Myxophobia
Small things	Microphobia Mycrophobia
Smells (and odours)	Olfactophobia Osmophobia Osphresiophobia
Snow	Chinophobia
Sourness	Acerophobia
Stars	Siderophobia
Stars (and celestial space)	Astrophobia
String	Linonophobia
Sun	Heliophobia
Symmetry (and symmetrical things)	Symmetrophobia
Thunder and lightning	Astraphobia Astrapophobla Brontophobia Ceraunophobia Keraunophobia Tonitrophobia
Tornadoes and hurricanes	Lilapsophobia
Trees	Dendrophobia
Vegetables	Lachanophobia
Voids (and empty spaces)	Kenophobia
Water (as in rabies)	Hydrophobia

Waves (and wavelike motions)	Cymophobia Kymophobia
Whirlpools (and dizziness)	Dinophobia
White (and white things)	Leukophobia
Wind	Ancraophobia Anemophobia
Wine	Oenophobia
Wooded areas (and forests at night)	Nyctohylophobia
Yellow (and yellow things)	Xanthophobia

Acrophobia

Ah heights! A fear of which is one of the most common phobias and one that by now you realise I have some insight on. If you haven't seen it, I can't recommend Alfred Hitchcock's *Vertigo* (1958) enough and even if you know it, why not go back and see it again. James Stewart plays John 'Scottie' Ferguson, a police officer who has to retire on seeing a fellow cop fall to his death. His reaction to heights is so extreme that he can't even stand on a stool without experiencing the symptoms of vertigo; dizziness, nausea, panic, profuse sweating etc.

Mention, of course, must also be made of the amazing dream sequence, devised by Surrealist master, Salvador Dali and still not bettered in its use of subconscious symbolism, although in essence *Vertigo* is not a film about one man's phobia, but rather obsession, of which the phobia is merely one strand.

In a recent interview, modern master Martin Scorsese nailed-down the film's dominant motif, 'Hitchcock's film is about obsession, which means that it's about circling back to the same moment, again and again. Which is probably why there are so many spirals and circles in the imagery ….' Ferguson's acrophobia may be only one strand of his tormented psyche, but

Hitchcock was wise enough to know that it stands as a metaphor for his whole character, the powerlessness and self-loathing and recriminations.

Eosophobia

Who would be eosophobic? Well of course vampires start to burn and eventually turn to dust when exposed to the first rays of dawn, but flying in the face of all the evidence (I've seen most episodes of 'Buffy ...') I've been assured they don't exist.

Most people see daybreak as full of the hope and promise of a new day, after the cold, dark terrors that night can instil. For many, days of religious significance logically use dawn as a signifier, especially when concerning fasts and fasting.

But the countdown to dawn can be tortuous; consider the condemned man awaiting execution or perhaps an army waiting for an attack.

Blood, injections and injury

Airborne substances (and draughts)	Aerophobia Ancraophobia Anemophobia
Being dirty	Automysophobia
Contamination with germs or dirt	Misophobia Molysmophobia Mysophobia Rupophobia
Contracting poliomyelitis	Poliosophobia
Definite disease	Monopathophobia
Diabetes	Diabetophobia
Disease	Nosophobia Pathophobia
Drugs (and taking them)	Pharmacophobia
Germs	Spermatophobia Spermophobia Verminophobia
Injections	Trypanophobia
Leprosy	Leprophobia Lepraphobia
Lues (and syphilis)	Luiphobia
Mercurial medicines	Hydrargyophobia
Needles (and pointed objects)	Aichmophobia Belonephobia Belonophobia
New drugs	Neopharmaphobia

Pins	Enetephobia Enetophobia Eretephobia
Points (differs from needles as can include anything from a mountain summit to a witches' hat)	Aichurophobia
Poisons (and being poisoned)	Iophobia Toxicophobia Toxiphobia Toxophobia
Rabies	Hydrophobia Hydrophobophobia
Radiation (and X-rays)	Radiophobia
Suffering (and disease)	Panthophobia Pathophobia
Surgery	Ergasiophobia Tomophobia
Syphilis	Syphilophobia
Vaccinations	Vaccinophobia

Phobias of needles and injections

According to a recent article, around 20% of Britons are scared of injections. Given that they hurt, no matter what the nice nurse tells you, that's hardly a big surprise. But a fully-fledged phobia of injections is something else, and serious, even deadly – it could easily prevent sufferers seeking life-saving treatment. Fear of injections is sometimes part of a wider phobia that extends to hospitals, doctors and all medical procedures. In much the same way, it's possible that the fear of injections lies behind other phobias of needles, pins, pointed things and sharp objects in general.

Most of us experience our first injections as children when we get our inoculations. No one can tell me they have fond memories of this. When you're a kid, needles are that much bigger: not just in our minds and our expectations of the pain they inflict, but really, truly huge. Remember how thin your arms were as a child? Didn't you believe that a hypodermic needle could go all the way through, given a tiny nudge?

Then of course there are dentists, where an injection is never an end in itself but merely the portent of exquisite tortures to come. Nothing compares to the scrape and crunch of steel penetrating bone, especially when it happens in your face. Then the white-hot needle twists in your jaw like a javelin wielded by a dervish. Makes your teeth ache just thinking about it.

But while some of us would do almost anything to avoid putting ourselves at the mercy of a needle, others seem quite content to endure the experience if they think it will make them look better. The growth in the body-modification market, be it tattooing, piercing, implants or just good old Botox, means that injections have become yet another tool that people use in the quest for beauty. For some, we can surmise, it's the transgressive nature of the act of injecting that provides part of the thrill.

Situations

Airsickness	Aeronausiphobia
Automobiles	Motorphobia
Being locked in an enclosed space	Cleisiophobia Cleithrophobia Clithrophobia
Bicycles	Cyclophobia
Carriages	Amakaphobia
Closeness to high buildings (and heights)	Batophobia
Confined spaces	Claustrophobia
Crossing bridges	Gephydrophobia Gephyrophobia Gephysrophobia
Crossing streets	Agyrophobia Dromophobia
Flying	Aviatophobia Aviophobia Pteromerhanophobia
Flying (and air)	Aerophobia
Glaring lights	Photoaugliaphobia
Glass	Hyalophobia Hyelophobia Nelophobia
Glass-bottomed things	Hyalinopygophobia
Looking up	Anablephobia

Mirrors (and seeing oneself in them)	Catoptrophobia Eisoptrophobia
Missiles (and bullets)	Ballistophobia
Narrowness	Anginophobia
Riding in a car (or other vehicle)	Amaxophobia
Road travel	Hodophobia
Ruins	Atephobia
Speed	Tachophobia
Stairs (and falling down them)	Climacophobia
Stairs (and steep slopes)	Bathmophobia
Trains and train travel	Siderodromophobia
Vehicles	Ochophobia

Catoptrophobia and Eisoptrophobia

Don't know about you, but I've never liked looking in mirrors. Since adolescence and the first (few!) spots, I've never been particularly happy with my reflection. We can safely speculate that at a basic level a fear of mirrors may have something to do with anxiety over our self-image. Do I really look like that? How long have I had those rings under my eyes? Where did those lines come from? Best not look too closely ...

I suspect there's a lot more to it than that, though. As a child, I found that mirrors conjured up a sense of vague unease. What if I look in the mirror and it shows something that isn't there. At an early age we learn that, in fact, mirrors don't reflect reality at all; the fun-fair mirror distorts and disturbs us while Alice's adventures *'Through the Looking-glass'*, (1896) introduce the notion that the mirror is in fact a portal to strange lands (let's face it, it's not as mundane as a wardrobe).

Prophecy involving staring into reflections (including water and polished surfaces as well as mirrors) is known as *scrying* and was the preferred method of divination for perhaps the greatest English mystic, Dr. John Dee (1527–1608.) Something of this sinister use of mirrors is present in the story of *'Snow White'*, and is quoted as recently as *Shrek* (2001) which, again,

111

we're exposed to and expose our own children to at a very early age; it's perhaps surprising that we ever look in them.

One of the defining images of twentieth century painting is Rene Magritte's *La Reproduction Interdite* ('Not to be Reproduced' (1937)), where we see the back of the head of one of Magritte's numerous petty bureaucrats. The man, gazing at his reflection, sees only his back reflected. What's it all mean? Mark Larabee, citing critic Cesare Casarino, says the painting 'illustrates the breakdown of subjectivity, the erasure of the face ....' It certainly seems to be some sort of meditation on the facelessness and mass-production of capitalist culture and perhaps the melancholic self-realisation of a lonely and isolated individual that he is literally 'not to be reproduced.' Rather than opening up a world of infinite possibility, the mirror here 'closes down', sucking in light and hopes like a black hole.

In film, mirrors often function in a similar way to that of labyrinths in mythology; a confusing and dangerous path to the centre of the villain's lair; think of the archetypal myth of Theseus and the Minotaur. The use of mirrors, of course, also makes for some great shots.

In *Enter the Dragon* (1973 dir. Robert Clouse), Bruce Lee's showdown with the evil Han (Kien Shih), takes place in a hall of mirrors as, only months later, did James Bond's (Roger Moore) with Francisco Scaramanga (Christopher Lee) in *The Man with the Golden Gun* (1974 dir. Guy Hamilton). Coincidence or tribute to the global phenomenon Bruce Lee had (posthumously) already become? Or perhaps merely testament to the enduring mystery of the humble mirror. In fact, both are probably tributes to/direct lifts from Orson Welles' *The Lady from Shanghai* (1948.)

I used to have the idea that if I looked in a mirror I would see the reflection of someone who has recently died. I can remember thinking this at quite a young age when I was first conscious of a death in my family. For a while I avoided looking in my bedroom mirror at all. I may even have covered it up.

Years later a close member of the family died while I was staying with my aunt and uncle. One of the rituals they observed was to cover every mirror in the house. I never asked why they did it but somehow formed the impression that it was connected with the belief that the spirit of the recently departed needs to leave the earthly realm as quickly as possible, and that mirrors might confuse or even trap it.

Indeed, the belief in a connection between mirrors and the soul has featured in many cultures. In his 1922 anthropological study *The Golden Bough*, Sir James Frazer notes that 'As some people believe a man's soul to be in his shadow, so other (or the same) peoples believe it to be in his reflection in water or a mirror.' Stories of tribes who believe that taking their photograph will rob them of their souls seem to belong to a similar tradition.

My mother has a more down-to-earth explanation for the covering of mirrors. She thinks it's simply to stop the bereaved being distracted by their own distress at a time when they have to cope not just with grief and loss but also with arranging the funeral and a host of other practical matters.

It's not as though we haven't been warned about the dangers of being obsessed by and absorbed into our own reflections. The myth of Narcissus (from which the term narcissism is obviously derived), has various variants, but whether the Roman version in which he falls, unknowingly, in love with his own reflection or the lesser-known Greek version in which he mistakes this reflection for that of his dead sister, both end with the beautiful youth's death, from thirst, rather than disturbing his beloved and watery reflection.

There must be something deeply arcane about mirrors; the breaking of no other household object carries seven years bad luck.

Episode 5:
Bruce Lee in a
bachelor flat

One of the interesting things about our sessions is that I can never predict what's going to happen. Using exactly the same patter from week to week, Ej gets an amazing range of different responses out of me.

Tonight we meet at his house. Unlike my cluttered shoe-box of a flat, it's spacious, tastefully decorated and – with a tired toddler padding around – a proper home. Perhaps that's the trouble: I'm out of my comfort zone.

I know the score now: the visualisation exercise, anchoring and then hypnosis. Ej asks me to imagine the party with my role model in attendance. This time, it feels different. For no apparent reason, I seem to have gone back 400 years: though it's still a party, there are Tudor costumes, long banqueting tables, lutes playing, elaborate paintings on the walls. First I see what look like Holbeins, then they turn to images of martyrs being burned, torture, burnings at the stake, flames and screaming.

Ej calms me down and tries the exercise from a different angle. We replace the party with a smaller dinner party. Now we're in a plush American bachelor flat and everything's friendly and funky again. Here's my role model looking cool and confident and poised (confession time: the man in question is none other than martial arts supremo Bruce Lee). Ice clunks in chunky tumblers of Scotch and soda; a cool album vamps quietly on the stereo. Not my normal scene by any means, but for now it's strangely comforting.

The frightful imagery earlier must have unsettled me, because things start to go wrong again. Whereas the previous week I'd got a huge buzz from Ej's talking me through my first Ramones gig, tonight I feel annoyed when he gets some of the details wrong. But why shouldn't he? It's my memory, not his. This is me being spiky, wanting other people to be perfect, getting exasperated at their mistakes. This is where I wallow in the perverse satisfaction that I'm about to be disappointed and let down yet again.

Do I sleep through the third part of our session or does it just feel like that? I've come to expect our evenings together to leave me feeling upbeat and relaxed. Tonight has been troubling. It's a relief to be slowly counting down from three hundred and beginning to drift.

Tomorrow we're going back to the library.

Arts, sciences
and the body

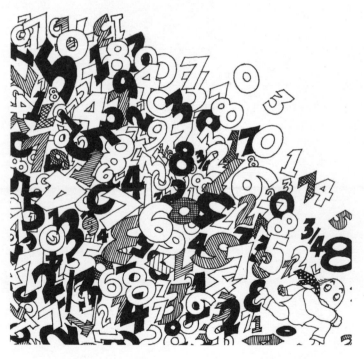

We put men on the moon, build super-colliders, anything to further mould the universe into a form we can understand, explain and (try to) dominate.

One would think that scientific progress would make us more rational and banish fears, but we all know now that's far from the case. By now you've probably realised, phobias are about the control, or rather the lack of it, we feel when confronted with the object of our terror. They're about what we find alien and intimidating. A blogger, Shar X, has a neat theory, specifically concerning spiders, but relevant to this argument; 'we tend to like people who bear some sort of resemblance to ourselves ... so maybe we hate spiders and other creepy-crawlies because *they are so very different to the way humans look* (my italics).'

All the scientific progress in the world can't change this and despite his cute glowing finger (and heart), E.T. would've been lynched in seconds.

123

The arts and sciences

Atomic explosions	Atomosophobia
Books	Bibliophobia
Clocks	Chronomentrophobia Chronometrophobia
Duration	Chronophobia
Flutes	Aulophobia
Ideas	Ideophobia
Infinity	Apeirophobia
Knowledge	Epistemophobia Gnosiophobia
Long words	Hippopotomonstrosesquip-pedaliophobia Sesquipedalophobia
Machines	Mechanophobia
Man-made satellites (and falling)	Keraunothnetophobia
Music	Melophobia Musicophobia
Myths (and stories)	Mythophobia
Nuclear weapons	Nucleomituphobia
The number 8	Octophobia
Numbers	Arithmophobia Numerophobia
Philosophy	Philosophobia
Poetry	Metrophobia

Scientific terms	Hellenologophobia
Symbolism	Symbolophobia
Technology	Technophobia
Time	Chronophobia
Words	Logophobia Verbophobia

Aulophobia

In a world full of musical instruments, why is the poor old flute singled out as an object of fear? Think of the damage that a beginner at the violin can do. And what about bagpipes?

I can only hope that the term aulophobia was coined to do justice to someone's deep aversion to Jethro Tull, or should it be Peter Gabriel-era Genesis? In fact when I think about it the entire late 60s/early 70s sound of Prog (progressive) Rock was characterised by these shrill sounds; Traffic, King Crimson, Moody Blues et al, all had flutes to the fore as did the Folk Rock scene. I'm sure phobias could have been formed at these gigs; bad vibes, bad drugs, hippies and interminable solos.

Or perhaps aulophobia taps into deeper reservoirs of fear. The flute signifies control; think of snake charmers and the myth of the Pied Piper, whose influence, though starting with rats, swiftly scaled-up to human children. No other instrument (except perhaps the Devil's alleged virtuosity on the fiddle) is so associated with power and dominion.

Perhaps, as with clowns, this phobia has older, even, pagan roots. One only needs to think of Pan and his ever-attendant pipes. The flute, like the ringmaster's cane, magician's wand or physician's caduceus, seems to belong to the order of phallic-objects of power, for which I must apologise to more sensitive readers.

Octophobia

And why, of all the numbers, is it 8 that has its very own phobia name? It seems innocuous enough – nothing 666 or 13-like about it. I genuinely can't find a root for this fear *unless* it has connections with a fear of eight-legged creatures, in which case it might be similar to arachnophobia or perhaps a fear of octo-puses and all octopods, which, significantly, doesn't appear to have a name.

My aversion to eight-legged creatures is currently spear-headed by the British 4x100m relay team which brings me nicely onto the Chinese, to whom the num-ber 8 is not only *not* to be feared, but incredibly lucky.

The 2008 Olympics not only started on August 8th (08/08/08) but at 8 minutes and 8 seconds past 8 (pm, local time). The criterion for a number's auspi-cious (or inauspicious) nature is based on its similarity to other Chinese words, (words of different meanings but that sound similar are called homophones).

Ironically both 13 and 666 are considered lucky to the Chinese; thirteen sounds similar to the words for imperatives *will* and *should* and so is seen as guarding against uncertainty and inaction, while 666 is sought after as a mobile-phone number and number plate, its homophone suggesting notions of flow and slipping and therefore seen as signifying that everything's going smoothly.

In the case of eight, its Chinese name *ba* is close enough to the word for wealth that it's always been linked to notions of prosperity, so much so that I've seen varying stories that the telephone number 8888-8888 sold, some years ago, for up to US$300,000.

Of course the Chinese government wouldn't give any credence to this superstition, preferring rather to announce that the games had to start sometime 'so why not respect the people's feelings.'

The body

Despite the classifications this book employs, it should be obvious by now that not only do some phobias 'float' between several categories but that to try to divide them between 'the physical' and, say, 'the emotional', is highly contentious; how, for instance, could a phobia *not* be both physical and emotional in terms of its origins and impact.

Of all things, an online guide to screenwriting gives us this alternative four-point guide to fears:

1. Fear of ourselves (most social phobias and those that I here call 'The Body' and 'Emotional' fall into this category.
2. Fear of those around us (see the 'people' category).
3. Fear of events around us ('Nature', 'Injury' and 'Situations').
4. Fear of the unknown (see 'Religion and Superstition').

Listed below are those phobias pertaining to ourselves, both as physical and conscious beings.

Amnesia	Amnesiphobia
Angina and choking	Anginophobia
Beards	Pogonophobia
Becoming ill	Nosemaphobia Nosophobia
Being contagious	Tapinophobia
Being dirty	Automysophobia
Blindness	Scotomaphobia
Blood	Haematophobia Hemaphobia Hemophobia Hematophobia
Brain disease	Meningitophobia
Cancer	Cancerphobia Cancerophobia Carcinophobia
Chins	Geniophobia
Choking and being smothered	Pnigerophobia Pnigophobia
Clothing	Vestiphobia
Decaying matter	Seplophobia
Deformity	Dysmorphophobia
Double vision	Diplophobia
Erect penises	Ithyphallophobia Medorthophobia Phallophobia
Eyes	Ommetaphobia Ommatophobia

Faecal matter	Coprophobia Scatophobia
Female genitalia	Eurotophobia
Fever	Febriphobia Fibriphobia Fibriophobia Pyrexiophobia
Genitals (particularly female)	Kolpophobia
Growing old	Gerascophobia
Hair	Chaetophobia Hypertrichophobia Trichopathophobia Trichophobia
Hands	Chirophobia
Heart conditions	Cardiophobia
Immobility of a joint	Ankylophobia
Injury	Traumatophobia
Kidney disease	Albuminurophobia
Knees	Genuphobia
Menstruation	Menophobia
Movement (and motion)	Kinesophobia Kinetophobia
Moving (and making changes)	Tropophobia
Muscular in-coordination	Ataxiophobia
Nosebleeds	Epistaxiophobia
Opening one's eyes	Optophobia

Pain	Agliophobia Algophobia
Painful bowel movements	Defecaloesiophobia
Pellagra	Pellagrophobia
Rabies	Kynophobia
Rectum and rectal diseases	Proctophobia Rectophobia
Scabies	Scabiophobia
Scratches and being scratched	Amychophobia
Semen	Spermatophobia
Shock	Hormephobia
Sitting down and being idle	Cathisophobia Kathisophobia
Skin and skin diseases	Dermatosiophobia Dermatophobia Dermatopathophobia
Standing and walking	Ambulophobia Stasibasiphobia Stasiphobia Stasophobia
Standing, walking and falling	Basiphobia Basophobia
Stooping	Kyphophobia
Swallowing, eating and being eaten	Phagophobia

Taste	Geumaphobia Geumatophobia Geumophobia
Teeth (and dental surgery)	Odontophobia
Tetanus (and lockjaw)	Tetanophobia
The heart	Cardiophobia
The left side of the body (and things to...)	Levophobia Sinistrophobia
The right side of the body (and things to...)	Dextrophobia
Touch	Haptophobia
Touching	Haphephobia Thixophobia
Trembling	Tremophobia
Trichinosis	Trichinophobia
Tuberculosis	Phthisiophobia Tuberculophobia
Urine and urinating	Urophobia
Venereal diseases (and prostitutes)	Cyprianophoia Cypridophobia Cyprinophobia Cypriphobia
Vomiting	Emetophobia
Walking	Ambulophobia Basophobia
Washing and bathing	Ablutophobia
Wet dreams	Oneirogmophobia
Wrinkles	Rhytiphobia

Episode 6: Carpet on the staircase

Spring has arrived, but so has winter (again). One day blizzard, the next drinking-on-the-prom scorchathon. Today is warm and sunny. I'm sitting outside the library not thinking about my ascent. Don't give the phobia any fuel. Attention feeds fear. Maybe Ej's methods have worked; at any rate, the idea I might be scared of walking up two flights of stairs seems absurd.

Ej arrives and we go in. I'm standing at the foot of the stairs. The library is quiet and cool. So am I. That's strange: the staircase in front of me has changed. It's shorter than I remember, and not so steep. The steel framework has been filled in and carpeted. That's not right. What's going on here?

It dawns on me that my mind has been playing tricks on me. My mental image of the staircase bears no resemblance to what I'm seeing. Yet it is so convincing that I have never doubted it. Nor has Ej. In our discussions, the staircase is the same creaking metal structure that Fletch climbed in Porridge. *Neither of us has ever looked closely at the real thing.*

Now that I have, walking up a wide carpeted staircase is easy. The only hiccup is when I glimpse light through the narrowest of gaps. My mind fills in the rest: an unfathomable drop waiting to claim its next victim. I take several deep breaths, think of Bruce Lee, run my Ramones soundtrack and walk with calm measured steps up the dozen or so steps to the landing.

Not that it's all easy. Passing someone on the stairs involves letting go of one handrail to clutch another. I'm momentarily thrown, but deal with it. The second flight is more difficult as I try to banish the fear that greater height means greater danger. I know that's not true and reason it out with Ej. We stand on the next landing and look around. I keep hold of the rail for comfort. It's too soon for complacency.

The descent is a breeze. I'm relieved to be back at ground level, but not overwhelmingly so; this time, the experience hasn't been traumatic. I'm delighted that I seem to have broken what I now see as just another bad habit.

Emotions and philosophy

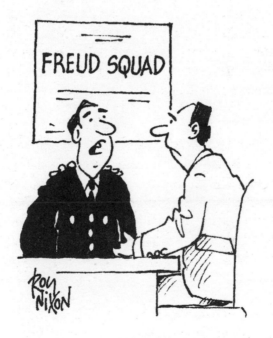

'TELL ME ABOUT YOUR FEAR OF POLICEMEN.'

Are we as humans the only species anxious enough to have phobias?

What about your bat, cat or (even) mole rat?

Some work's been done on studying these responses in dogs, whose phobias mainly comprise those to do with noise and place. The phobic condition means that these fearful circumstances don't lose their potency over time or through exposure.

The physical symptoms will include increased heart rate and sweating (expressed through panting), similar to humans and a possible loss of control of urinary and defecating functions, hopefully dissimilar to most humans.

They may exhibit the same 'fight or flight' reactions as humans and these will depend on many factors. It's safe to say the same old 'nature versus nurture' argument means each case has to be assessed independently. An animal behaviourist might be a good bet as many dog owners make the (apparent) mistake of rewarding their pets for facing their fears, which might actually serve to reinforce the phobic reaction in the future.

Changes	Metathesiophobia
Cheerfulness	Cherophobia
Disorder	Ataxiophobia
Dreams	Oneirophobia
Duration	Chronophobia
Everything	Panophobia Panphobia Pantophobia
Feeling pleasure	Hedonophobia
Freedom	Eleutherophobia
Gaiety	Cherophobia
Heredity	Patroiophobia
Ideas	Ideophobia
Illness	Nosemaphobia
Imperfection	Atelophobia
Insanity	Agateophobia Dementophobia Lyssophobia (from rabies Maniaphobia
Jealousy	Zelophobia
Justice	Dikephobia
Knowledge	Gnosiophobia
Many things	Polyphobia
Materialism (and epilepsy)	Hylephobia
Memories	Mnemophobia
Monotony	Homophobia

New things (and ideas)	Cainophobia Caintophobia Cenophobia Centophobia Kainolophobia Kainophobia Neophobia
Overworking (and pain)	Ponophobia
Pain	Algophobia Odynephobia Odynophobia
Phobias	Phobophobia
Pleasure	Hedonophobia
Progress	Prosophobia
Shock	Hormephobia
The mind	Psychophobia
Thinking	Phronemophobia
Ugliness	Cacophobia
Untidiness	Ataxophobia
Wealth	Plutophobia
Work	Ergophobia
Working, functioning and operating	Ergasiophobia

Miscellaneous

In the darkest hinterland of life in the early twenty-first century nothing is above being worthy of our fears. Look at the ramshackle bunch below; it reads like a desk sergeant's inventory of the contents of Bill Sykes' pockets.

In fact as I've probably commented before, we're notoriously conservative in our fears, even superstitious (as I'll show) and our fears are often anachronistic. We simply aren't keeping up with the changes in society. As Öhman and Mineka put it 'We are more likely to fear events and situations that provided threats to the survival of our ancestors, such as potentially deadly predators, heights and wide open spaces, than to fear the most frequently encountered potentially deadly objects in our contemporary environment, such as weapons or motorcycles.'

Buttons	Koumpounophobia
Fabrics	Textophobia
Money	Chrometophobia Chrematophobia
Knives	Aichmophobia
Property	Orthophobia
Razors	Xyrophobia

Koumpounophobia

Ah, the humble, honest button; who could possibly be scared of these?

Actually it seems to be a fairly common phobia, at least in my admittedly limited experience. I know three sufferers, all women in their late 30s and early 40s who are affected to varying degrees. Does this reflect some post-war golden age of button use in the 60s and 70s before Velcro muscled in? (No, let's be honest, it's more likely to be because most of the people I know are around that age.)

The symptoms are remarkably consistent: none of the three can wear clothes with buttons, nor can they handle buttons or even say the word 'button' without anxiety.

Indeed, one of them almost gagged when she tried. Maybe this is another phobia that can be explained by childhood misadventure? Did our subjects nearly choke on buttons as toddlers, leaving them with an aversion so deep as to give rise to a phobia of the name as well as the object?

In the press, I was able to find only one sufferer of a button phobia, and guess what, she's a woman in her thirties. Sarah Barker's phobia didn't concern buttons on her clothes, but those on sofas, chairs and mattresses: 'I couldn't bear them to touch my skin and would scream for them to be kept away from me. My dad told me to stop being silly and my mum thought it was just a phase.'

Left untreated, Sarah's phobia soon turned from anxiety about buttons to avoidance and flight from them. It cost her jobs, relationships and a social life until she sought hypnotherapy. She discovered that her fear had had a very specific trigger. While at a sleepover at a friend's house at the age of seven, 'a glass jar had fallen from a shelf and landed next to my head. The loud noise scared me and I started to cry ... I could hardly sleep afterwards.' The article didn't state whether Sarah was also scared of sudden noises – fireworks, balloons bursting, lightning, breaking glass – but I would hazard a guess that she probably was. I have no way of knowing if my three phobics shared any pivotal experience similar to this; two I knew before this project and merely thought it a strange coincidence. The third thinks buttons remind her of gravy and old ladies (though whether that's together, I'm not wholly sure).

Fortunately, though, Sarah's story has a happy ending. After only four sessions of hypnotherapy she was able to brave John Lewis's bed department on her own. That's some achievement.

Episode 7: Alone at the library

Agreeing to take an evening off, Ej and I go to a gig. Unlike our previous meeting places, the club is loud and I'm uncomfortable. The night is not a success and I apologise to Ej afterwards for my bad mood. He suggests I take myself back to the library, climb up to the second-floor balcony and pat myself on the back.

So I get myself ready, set off and swagger like Bruce Lee through the surrounding streets. Once I'm outside the library my heart starts to race. I put it down to the excitement of expectation, not fear. Inside I don't recognise any of the friendly faces that we've briefed about the project. I ask a librarian for permission to photograph; she's not sure and points towards a couple of maintenance men.

I feel small. For a moment my request and the whole endeavour seem pointless. It was so much easier when Ej was here.

I tap my face rapidly – the secret trigger that unleashes the power of my Ramones memory. I assure the janitors that I'm only interested in filming the staircase, not the people around us (do I look like some kind of pervert?), and I'm off.

I bound purposefully up the first flight, not even holding the handrail. It's surprisingly easy now I've finally been persuaded the structure is safe. Those pesky glimmers of depths between stair and wall catch me out again but I know I can't fall and banish the fear without any trouble. The second flight makes me more anxious and I seek solace from the handrail for the last few steps.

Done! I pause at the top landing to take in the building, where I am and what I've achieved. Little victories ...

I descend, if not exactly exultant, then certainly satisfied at what we've achieved so far.

Religion and
superstition

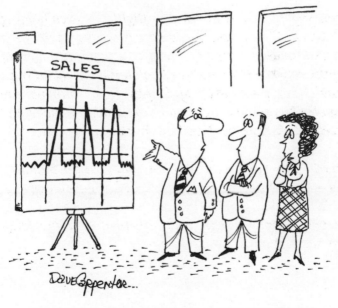

'I'M NOT SUPERSTITIOUS EITHER, BUT THOSE WERE THE
THREE DAYS HARRIS WORE HIS LUCKY SOCKS.'

cartoonstock.com

Harvard University's Kevin Foster thinks that 'the tendency to falsely link cause to effect – a superstition – is occasionally beneficial.' The argument given is of a prehistoric man associating the sound of rustling grass with the advance of a hostile predator and so hiding or taking flight. Although more often than not it's merely the wind causing this phenomenon, our early man will react each time as though it's potentially the worst case scenario; a primitive (and unconscious) version of the old 'better safe than sorry' mantra. Or as a paper for the Psychological Review more succinctly puts it 'In the early mammalian environment of evolutionary adaptiveness, disaster could strike fast and without warning, primarily through hunting predators but also through aggressive conspecifics and from physical events such as falling objects, floods, thunder and lightning and sudden lack of Oxygen. Escape and avoidance were common strategies designed by evolution to deal with such exigencies.'

This begs the question as to why superstitions don't become redundant as the real dangers they represent become further removed from us in time. Our aforementioned Professor Foster believes that people would rather carry on with an outmoded superstition than think they might miss something or be 'tempting fate'; a bit like a committed lottery player not daring to miss a week for the fear (nay, certainty) their numbers would come up that one time or forgetting to cross your fingers in a situation and then when things go wrong, blaming your own negligence.

It's not just religious superstitions Foster criticises but pretty much the whole 'New Age' phenomenon itself including Alternative Medicine and Homeopathy, seeing most of it as ineffective and actually blaming science's methodology of linking cause and effect; 'Science is simply a dogmatic form of superstition' and indeed recently this has been a charge levelled at 'arch-atheist' Richard Dawkins, especially in the more agnostically-inclined pages of *Fortean Times*.

Crosses and crucifixes	Staurophobia Stigiophobia Stygiophobia
Demons	Daemonophobia Demonophobia
Friday the 13th	Paraskavedekatriaphobia
God and gods	Theophobia Zeusophobia
Halloween	Samhainophobia
Heaven	Ouranophobia Uranophobia
Hell	Hadephobia
Sacred things	Hierophobia
Spectres and ghosts	Phasmophobia Spectrophobia
Spirits	Pneumatiphobia
The number 13	Terdekaphobia Triskaidekaphobia
The number 616	Hexakosioidekahexaphobia
The number 666	Hexakosioihexekontahexaphobia
Theology	Theologicophobia
Tombstones	Placophobia

Terdekaphobia/Triskaidekaphobia

Supposedly the most widespread phobia in America, fear of the number 13 is far older and widespread than its place within the Christian pantheon of phobias and superstitions might suggest.

To put its pre-eminence into context, a Google search for 'Religion + Superstition + Phobias' will throw back nearly 12,000 hits, add 'Friday 13th' and you're left with barely a dozen (irony intended!).

Apparently 13 has always been thought of strange and sinister. Other than decimal, (and obviously pre-binary), 12 is the commonest counting base. Pre-decimal British currency had 12 pennies to the shilling and goods were commonly packaged in dozens (12) and grosses (12 x 12/144.) I remember at school learning and reciting tables, but only up to 12. As I said, 13 represents unknown territory; the Tarot card for *Death* is numbered 13, though I'm told this is symbolic of transformation and not to be taken too literally.

If most people were asked to say why 13 is considered so unlucky, to the point where some houses, flats and floors of buildings won't use the number, they'd probably cite the 13 present at the Last Supper (Jesus + 12 disciples), but this notion of the unluckiness of any gathering of 13 also has parallels in Ancient Egyptian, Hindu and Viking culture.

Unfortunately the Apollo 13 disaster, in 1970, lent further credence to this superstition. The almost fatal disaster happened at 13.13 on April 13th, which is now deemed 'International Phobia Day' (although I would argue this disaster has, in reality, nothing to do with any real phobia.)

Hexakosioihexekontahexaphobia

'Here is wisdom. Let him that hath understanding count the number of the beast: for it is the number of a man; and his number is six hundred threescore and six.'
The Revelation of St John the Divine, 13:18

Like most of the items featured in our list of religious phobias, the fear of the number 666 has Biblical roots. Unlike most of the other phobias, though, it seems to be on the increase as more and more people see the political and religious turmoil in today's world as a portent of approaching apocalypse.

In contrast to other major monotheistic religions such as Judaism, Islam and the Baha'i faith, Christianity includes within it the idea of powerful supernatural enemies of God and embodiments of evil: the Antichrist, the Beast (666) and the devil or Satan. The need to explain the existence of evil in a world supposedly created and governed by a good and all-powerful God has always been a source of theological difficulty. Since Zoroastrianism the idea of some form of devil (often an angel who has fallen from grace after threatening God's supremacy) has been incorporated into various forms of doctrine to give believers an explanation as to how the world came to be in its imperfect condition.

Wholly at odds with the rest of the New Testament, which concerns Christ's life and mission and the lives and epistles of the apostles after His death, The Revelation of St John the Divine is hallucinatory in feel, and obscured by deep symbolism. As the last book of the Bible, it stands as a counterpoint to the first, Genesis, with its account of how God created the world in six (he rested on the seventh, remember?), days. Some people choose to interpret the Bible as an entire history of the world and God's plan for it from creation to eventual destruction.

But what does 666 represent, and why is it so feared by the many millions of Christians who inhabit cyberspace? When I checked, there were in excess of

100 million Internet references to 666, many of which were concerned with the last days of Biblical prophecy. Revelations aside, the number 666 had a fairly undistinguished past; it was the number of gold talents King Solomon collected in a year and the number of Adonikam's descendants who returned from captivity in Babylon. In Kabbalah, the Jewish form of mysticism, the number 666 is sometimes held to be mystical and holy, and may represent the physical universe.

Religious associations aside, 666 has its own fascinations in purely numerical terms. To me, its notation in Greek looks like a beast (possibly slouching towards Bethlehem): χξϛ′. Some commentators have made much of the fact that it is the sum of the first six Roman numerals: I + V + X + L + C + D. A mathematician called Mike Keith proclaims that 'The number 666 is cool' and then goes to prove it by presenting nine pages featuring dozens of mathematical formulae all involving this sinister and elusive number. For beginners, 666 is an abundant, palindromic, repdigit, triangular and Smith number and the sum of the squares of the first seven prime numbers. (Any number that has 666 digits is called an apocalypse number.) Mike Keith ends on a cautionary note; 'If the letter A is defined to be equal to 36 (6 x 6), B = 37, C = 38 and so on, then the sum of the letters in the word SUPERSTITIOUS is 666.'

In popular culture, the number 666 has been appro-priated by the heavy metal brigade. There's hot debate over who first put black magic into metal – among the chief suspects, Jimmy Page of Led Zeppelin's obsession with Aleister Crowley, while Black Sabbath were more inclined towards Dennis Wheatley and Hammer Horror – but a good many metal bands liked to present themselves as dabblers in the occult. Iron Maiden's 1982 breakthrough album was entitled *The Number of the Beast*, exposing the band to charges of Satanism, though the band's bassist and writer Steve Harris claimed his inspiration came from nightmares (another recurring rock motif adopted by Alice Cooper and Metallica among many others). A sub-genre, 'Black-metal', has been described as a ter-rifying mix of 'Satanism, neo-paganism and National Socialism ... the most extreme form of underground music on the planet' and has been held responsible for the burning down of churches and murder. But apocalyptic themes aren't confined to the metal brigade: post-punk band Killing Joke explores 666 and all it stands for in its albums *Revelations* (1982) and *Killing Joke* (2003).

The Vatican takes the interest in Satanism and all aspects of the occult so seriously that it plans to train hundreds of priests as exorcists and reinstate a prayer to the Archangel St Michael as a 'sort of DIY demon-buster for the ordinary believer.'

But maybe the hexakosioihexekontahexaphobic should relax: not everyone is convinced that the number of the Beast is actually 666. Let's look at the other contenders. An early variant from the eleventh century is 665, though it may have been a misprint and didn't really catch on. But 616 really got the Biblical scholars going. It derives from the most important find in the history of Revelation scholarship, a 1,700-year-old papyrus that was discovered, like its better-known predecessor the Dead Sea Scrolls, among discarded rubbish, this time in the city of Oxyrhynchus in Egypt.

The job of translating the papyrus fell to a research team from the University of Birmingham led by David Parker, a professor of palaeography and New Testament textual criticism. It turned out to be the earliest known transcription of the Book of Revelation and cites the number of the Beast as 616. Professor Parker suggests that this is a reference to the Roman emperor Caligula, whose name in Greek and Hebrew can be calculated as having the numerical value 616. Among the many atrocities and outrages that Caligula committed during his mercifully brief reign, he pronounced that he was a god and tried to have a statue of himself erected in the sacred temple in Jerusalem – both appalling blasphemies in the eyes of the early apostles and indeed of followers of the Jewish faith in general.

To those of a fundamentalist bent, the mark of the Beast is just as important as its number. A signifier of the Antichrist's dominion over the world, the mark of the Beast must be worn by all on either the right hand or the forehead. In what we might interpret as a peculiar strain of technophobia, some people regard modern tracking technologies as a mark of the Beast. One day, will we all have barcodes tattooed on us once credit has replaced cash and we're scanned along with our groceries? Let's not forget RFID (radio frequency identification) tags that broadcast their whereabouts and the sub-dermal micro-chipping sometimes done on cats and dogs, but maybe one day coming our way ...

These sorts of fear lead some people to believe that we are living through the end of the world and a jump-off point they call the rapture. Many of the websites concerned with these beliefs are repugnant in the extreme. Some carry warnings but I'll add my own: don't go there, I have, so you don't need to. Oh, just one more warning: don't plan any parties for Christmas or New Year's Eve 2012.

Stop press

I'm the world's biggest *Deal or No Deal* fan. (For anyone who doesn't know: it's a daytime TV competition presented by Noel Edmonds in which contestants have to choose from a number of boxes which contain cash prizes of different values ... oh, go and watch it, why don't you?) But one show was particularly memorable. On 26 March 2008, one of the randomly selected contestants was a priest who had been ordained in late middle age. Unlike many contestants, Reverend David professed to have no superstitions, lucky numbers or systems for picking the boxes, which he thought would be incompatible with his Christian faith.

Having chosen his first five boxes, Reverend David received his first offer from the Banker. Cue spooky music: said offer was for £666. The good reverend hastily declined, saying he'd do no deal with the devil. But from then on the whole game was spooked. Box 2, when opened, was empty. It should have contained one of the twenty-two cards showing the amount (from 1p to £250,000) that the contestant could win. There had never been an empty box in over 700 games and Noel Edmond's initial disbelief soon turned into dismay that he or the show might appear unprofessional.

The game had to be stopped while various options were considered. Once the remaining boxes had been reshuffled and resealed, play resumed. The previously empty box should have contained the top prize of £250,000 which has only ever been won once; people duly 'ooh'ed and 'aah'ed and in a show of solidarity the confetti, solely reserved for the big win, drifted down from the ceiling of its own accord.

The Reverend struck a deal early at £12,500, perhaps reconsidering the hastiness of his earlier diatribe against superstition.

Not impressed? I've seen many horror films with far flimsier premises.

Episode 8:
Climbing St Paul's

So here I am in London with Ej. He's determined we attempt to climb up the inside of St Paul's Cathedral; I'm just as determined we don't. The mere idea is terrifying.

Outside St Paul's, I marvel at the scale of it. I'm standing right outside and I can't even see the dome. Ej sees me flinch and takes me round the corner to a quieter spot. He talks me through the now familiar routines. I have trouble concentrating. We've always done this in a quiet room in the evening, but now all I can hear is traffic and children. Eventually my breathing starts to slow down and my nerves steady a little. I haven't even been thinking about the climb; I'm so preoccupied with getting away that I've forgotten why I am here.

'Ten pounds?' That's the cost of going up to the top. For a tenner I could drink six cans of Stella, eat a kebab and get

in a fight if I wanted to pay for the privilege of being sick and scared. Still, what's £10 after all we've been through?

It's actually hard to be scared of heights climbing St Paul's. The winding stone staircases and labyrinth of narrow wooden passages make the experience more like walking through a haunted house at a funfair. (Scary enough for some, I admit.) We come out into the whispering gallery and I suddenly feel faint.

We're barely a third of the way up and the nave and quire yawn like some beautiful crater below. The ground falls away and I sit with my back pressed into the stone behind me. I try to relax and tell myself it's as safe as sitting in my second-floor flat. But I feel as though I'm in a centrifuge. As a steady stream of tourists pour into the gallery, all the techniques I've been taught go out the window.

Back on the relative safety of the stairs, I grip a handrail and try not to panic. My fear level goes down a few notches. Throughout all this Ej says very little. This is my show. Although I want to leave, I know I've let myself down once this week already and tell Ej I want to try again. Cautiously, I step out into the gallery and sit down.

I make a conscious effort to remember how to breathe and relax. I invoke my role model (yo, Bruce) and my empowering memory of that Ramones gig. For the first time I look properly at this magnificent interior. It starts me off on a monologue about St Augustine and St Gregory and why the four evangelists are represented by creatures from the visions of Ezekiel. It's half-remembered trivia like this that keeps me going.

After my spiel I realise I'm tired and have had enough. Ej makes me focus on what we've achieved and reminds me to congratulate myself. A month ago, I couldn't climb two flights of stairs; now I've staggered up 163 steps and looked down from a height of 30 metres.

Getting to the top of the dome would have made for a neater ending, but that's not what happened. Even so, I feel much more positive, and tell myself I'll go back some day.

We decide to have one last session at Ej's, and try two new visualisation techniques.

The first involves taking note of where fear strikes and how it travels through my body. I need to visualise removing the fear and mentally turning this negative feeling into a positive one, a technique known as spinning the fear. In my case, fear enters through my legs, which buckle beneath me. It whips around my spine and I feel as though I'm being pushed backwards. The queasiness is like being seasick. Then I sense the fear trying to get out through my eyes. I feel winded but can't tear my eyes from the drop below.

Ej gets me to visualise taking the feeling out of my stomach and holding it like a ball in front of me. I'm to turn it through 180 degrees to make the negative positive, then spin it in my hands so fast I can feel the heat, before pushing it back, still spinning, into my stomach. It sounds ridiculous, but it works. What you're doing is robbing the phobia of its hold over you and turning fear into positive anticipation.

Now I'm ready for my second exercise. This is called swoosh pattern or swish movement, and seems to involve holding at least three different perspectives simultaneously. First, I am an actor on a screen playing out my confrontation with my phobia. Second, I am in the cinema audience watching this scene unfold. Third, I am the cinema projectionist, able to see and control both the screening of the film and the viewer's reactions.

Ej gets me to visualise my experience at St Paul's backwards, from reaching a point of relative comfort up in the gallery to the worst moment as I start out on the climb.

For once he tells me exactly what I'll see and how I'll see it. We run the memories like a black and white clip of some silent slapstick comedy, going faster and faster. The jumble of sights, sounds and emotions gets smaller and more insignificant. Then Ej catapults a brilliant Technicolor multiplex-sized print of the Ramones gig into my head. It wipes out the last vestiges of my fear.

164

For the third course, as usual, I'm hypnotised. All I have to do is lie down and fall asleep. No tiresome exercises, moments of self-doubt or self-realisation, just Ej's voice and some faraway music. How long does it take? I have no way of knowing – neither of us counts the time.

While Ej gets ready to drive me home, I sit and talk to his wife. For no apparent reason, I feel compelled to roll up my trousers. What a bizarre thing to do in front of someone I barely know. Then I get it.

Whenever my acrophobia strikes, my knees always buckle. It's that that makes me think I'm going to fall to my death. What I'm scared of is not danger itself, but the thought that I'm not up to dealing with it. Every time I feel anxious or inadequate, I get this sense of physical collapse.

Perhaps it was on an early trip to St Paul's, perhaps it was at some other high building, and it really doesn't matter. As I reached the top, the fatigue in my legs from climbing all those stairs, the burn from the build-up of lactic acid in my knees, must have kicked in and for a moment I must have thought my legs might give way. My acrophobia was born.

That explains why I was afraid of gaps I couldn't possibly fall through. It wasn't about falling, but failing.

My knees aren't going to give out and I'm not going to fall, or fail. I know that now.

Source notes

Introduction

What is a phobia?

The definitions at the beginning of this chapter are taken from *The New Collins Compact Dictionary of the English Dictionary* (HarperCollins, 1984), *Collins Cobuild Advanced Learner's English Dictionary* (HarperCollins, 1987), *Reader's Digest Family Guide to Alternative Medicine* (Reader's Digest, 1991, p. 276), *Collins Pocket Thesaurus* (HarperCollins, 1995) and I. M. Marks, *Fears and Phobias* (New York Academic Press, 1969).

'Anxious individuals inaccurately appraise ...' 'the face of the Greek god Phobos': Aaron T. Beck, *Anxiety Disorders and Phobias: A Cognitive Perspective* (Basic Books, 1985, pp. xvi and 115).

'The mode of being ...' Martin Heidegger (trans. Theodore Keisel), *History of the Concept of Time* (Indiana University Press, 1985, p. 284).

'I salute you, Isaac Marks and Paul Bebbington': I. M. Marks and P. Bebbington, 'Space phobia: syndrome or agoraphobic variant?' *British Medical Journal*, August 1976, Vol. 2. Issue 6031, pp. 345–7, quoted in Richard Stern, *Mastering Phobias* (Penguin, 1995).

'Phobic people ...': Stern, *Mastering Phobias,* p. 1.

Where do they come from?

'According to Dr Angharad Rudkin': quoted in Judy Yorke, 'Mummy, I'm scared!' *Daily Mirror*, 21 February 2008.

'One US study': Stern, *Mastering Phobias*, p. 8.

Young Hans: Stern, p. 12.

'As young children': quoted at www.phobialist.com/class.

Episode 1: My phobia and me

'I jumped out of plane to cure fear of heights,' Bill Gibb, *Weekly News*, 1 March 2008.

Self-help and other treatments

A health warning

'One well-respected guide': *Reader's Digest Family Guide to Alternative Medicine*, Reader's Digest, 1991, p. 277.

'As one phobia expert says': Aaron T. Beck, *Anxiety Disorders and Phobias*, p. 316.

Cognitive therapy

'Problem-solving techniques': Richard Stern, *Mastering Phobias*, p. 6.

'Ten principles': *Anxiety Disorders and Phobias*, p. 167.

'Being aware': *Anxiety Disorders and Phobias*, pp. 319–20.

'AWARE' etc.: *Anxiety Disorders and Phobias*, pp. 323–4.

Systematic desensitization

'Similar to "classical conditioning therapy" …' see 'Systematic desensitization' at en.wikipedia.org/wiki/Systematic_desensitization

Hypnotherapy

'In a recent TV programme ...' *Alternative Therapies: Hypnotherapy*, produced and directed by Nicola Stockley, BBC for the Open University, 2008.

'As Derren Brown says': in *Tricks of the Mind*, Channel 4 Books, 2007, p. 198.

Medication

'The role of medication': in *Mastering Phobias*, pp. 108–15.

Agoraphobia and social phobias

'Standard psychiatric categorisations': *Diagnostic and Statistical Manual of Mental Disorders*, 4th edition, American Psychiatric Association, Washington DC, 1995.

Agoraphobia

'This is one of the commonest ... 15 and 35': Richard Stern, 'How common are phobias?' *Mastering Phobias*, p. 7.

Social phobias

'One study found ...' Stern, 'Social Phobias', *Mastering Phobias*, p. 31.

Meat

'The average person ...' Robert Anton Wilson, *Prometheus Rising*, New Falcon Publications, 1983, p. 234.

'(Which is dubious)': see Edwin Moore, *Lemmings Don't Leap*, Chambers Harrap, 2006.

'As *Cuy* ... roast ... Guinea Pig is consumed ...' see www.deathby1000papercuts.com/peruvian-delicacy-of-cuy-dining-on-roasted-guinea-pig.

'Consider Nat Holland ... ' 'Pork life,' *Daily Mirror*, 9 February 2008.

'Chris Hawkins ...': in Bill Gibb, 'Fruit or veg made me feel like passing out,' *Weekly News*, 2 February 2008.

Animals, people, dummies and the like

'Those characterised by persistent and irrational fear ...' Although quoted verbatim at 60 Internet sites from www.everything2.com/title/phobia to www.megaes says.com/essay_search/persistent_fear.html I've found it impossible to find the original source.

Animals

'Certain objects may have a genetic predisposition ...' 'Phobias: Causes and Treatment in AllPsych Journal, www.allpsych.com/journal/phoias.html quoted at en.wikipedia.org/wiki/Phobia

'An unnatural or illogical functioning of the brain ...' see 'Phobia' at en.wikipedia.org/wiki/Phobia

Zemmiphobia

'Endowed with pinkish-grey, wrinkly skin ...' Jill Locantore, 'The truth about mole rats,' The Smithsonian's National Zoological Park site at www.nationalzoo.si.edu/Search/default.cfm.

People

'Homophobia is not a phobia ...' see planetout.com/news/article-print.html?2002/06/13/3.

Coulrophobia

'A clown can go anywhere ...': *These Foolish Things*, Jonathan Brown, Gerard Chen, Nicole Gallivan, Tiffany Rosheuvel and James Ward, graduation documentary, Goldsmiths College, University of London, 2007.

'There are no rules ...': *The Convention Crashers*, produced and directed by Will Yapp, Channel 4, 2008.

'When I was eight ...' 'Stories from you II,' www.clownz.com.

'A clown got right up ...': Alex Waterfield, 'Fear of clowns no laughing matter', Columbia News Service, 27 December 2005.

'I'd argued that many people's coulrophobia ...' '*Don't send in the Clowns: The Evil Clown*', *Fortean Times*: 226, August 2007, p. 36.

'Only Pennywise has an independent existence ...' Ibid.

'These moral panics ...' letters page, *Fortean Times*: 228, October 2007, p. 74.

'In a letter to *Fortean Times*' and 'the white face ...' letters page, *Fortean Times*: 228, October 2007, p. 75.

'Renders the observer ...': Kathryn Cillick, quoted at www.phobialist.com.

'Clowns by nature ...': Ann Keong, quoted in 'Stories for you II,' at www.clownz.com.

'All of them disliked clowns ...' and 'they don't look funny ...': Dave Sutton, 'Clowns are scary – it's official,' *Fortean Times*, 233, March 2008, p. 2.

Dummies and the like

'Everything that I think I can't say ...' and 'Keep them living ...' from *The Convention Crashers*, produced and directed by Will Yapp, Channel 4, 2008.

Techgnosis, Erik Davis, Three Rivers Press, 1998.

'Perhaps a corpse ...' from the author's introduction to the revised 1831 edition.

'Long-term sexual ...' Graeme Green, 'Not tonight, my dear ...' *Metro*, 16 April 2008.

'Men with low self-esteem ...' Dr Glyn Hudson-Allez, quoted in the article above.

'Joanna Eberhart ... not only finds ...' See *The Stepford Wives* entry on Wikipedia at en.Wikipedia.org/wiki/The_Stepford_Wives.

'They are coming ... ' from *Terminator: The Sarah Connor Chronicles*, 'The Demon Hand,' series 1 episode 7, Warner Bros, 2008.

'Point of singularity': the term comes from *Terminator*.

'According to one technology expert': Ray Kurzweil, quoted in Steve Connor, 'Computers to match human brains by 2030,' *The Independent*, 16 February 2008.

Nature, injury and situations

Acrophobia

'In a recent interview ...' 'The Best Music in Film' at www.bfi.org.uk/sightandsound/filmmusic/detail.php ?t=d&q=42

Phobias of needles and injections

'According to a recent article ...' Ron McManus, 'New treatment gets to the point of needle fear,' *Weekly News*, 16 February 2008.

Catoptrophobia and Eisoptrophobia

'Mark Larabee, citing critic Cesare Casarino ...' Mark D. Larabee *Modernity at Sea: Melville, Marx, Conrad in Crisis (review)* MFS Modern Fiction Studies, Volume 49, Number 4, Winter 2003, pp. 874–876. The Johns Hopkins University Press.

Arts, sciences and the body

'A blogger, Shar X ...' See 'Are you scared of spiders and if so, what is it about spiders that frightens you ...? at uk.answers.yahoo.com/question/index?qid=20080 829083522AAC3lyx

Octophobia

'The 2008 Olympics not only started …' See 'Numbers in Chinese Culture' at en.wikipedia.org/wiki/Numbers_in_Chinese_culture and 'Chinese counting on lucky number 8' at www.cnn.com/2008/WORLD/asiapcf/08/08/china.eight

'So why not respect the people' feelings …' See 'Chinese counting …' cited above.

The Body

'Of all things, an online guide to screenwriting …' See 'Defining characters by their fears' and 'Fears' at www.makemovies.co.uk/characters/page08htm

Emotions and philosophy

'Some work's been done…' see 'Fear and phobias in the dog: causes and solutions…' at www.vetontheweb.co.uk/pet-clinic-detail.asp?id=128

Miscellaneous

'As Öhman and Mineka put it …' see 'Fears, Phobias and Preparedness: Toward an Evolved Module of Fear and Fear Learning' by Arne Öhman and Susan Mineka. Psychological Review 2001, vol. 108, No. 3, pp. 483–522.

Koumpounophobia

'Sarah Barker's phobia ...' Debbie Marco, 'My fear of buttons made me feel like a freak,' *Sunday Mirror*, January 2008.

Religion and superstition

'Harvard University's Kevin Foster ...' see 'Has Superstition Evolved To Help Mankind Survive?' at www.science.slapshot.org/article.pl?sid=08/09/10/22 30253&from=rss

'In a paper for the Psychological Review ...' see source under **Miscellaneous** above.

'Science is simply a dogmatic form of superstition ...' see 'Has Superstition Evolved ...' cited above.

Terdekaphobia/Triskaidekaphobia

'Are You Superstitious? Friday the 13th' by Wenona Napolitano at www.associatedcontent.com/article/ 187685/are_you_superstitious_friday_the_13th.html

'Why are people afraid of the number 13? At www. funtrivia.com/askft/Ouestion2217.html (sic.) and

'Freaky Friday' at www.beliefnet.com/story/118/ story_11851_1.html

Hexakosioihexekontahexaphobia

'The number of gold talents King Solomon collected ...' 1 Kings 10:14 and 2 Chronicles 9:13.

'The number of Adonikam's descendants ...' Ezra 2:13.

'In Kabbalah ...' here and elsewhere in the section, I'm drawing on Wikipedia.

'One online commentator proclaims ...' Mike Keith, 'The number of the Beast' at users.aol.com/s6sj7gt/mike666.html.

'There's hot debate ...'and 'Satanism, neo-paganism and National Socialism ...' see Michael Moynihan and Didrik Soderland, *Lords of Chaos*, Feral House, 1998.

'Sort of DIY demon-buster ...' 'War on Satan hots up,' *Fortean Times*, 233, March 2008.

'But 616 really got the biblical scholars going ...' acknowledgement and thanks must here be given to the scholarly *QI* team and their *Book of General Ignorance*.

'Don't plan any parties ...': www.satansrapture.com.

Useful links

Not everyone is lucky enough to have access to a hypnotherapist. People wanting to know more about phobias should find these websites a good place to start (but beware, you enter them at your own risk).

www.achildinmind.co.uk
www.anxietymatters.com
www.changes.co.uk
www.changethatsrightnow.com
www.findhypnotherapist.com
www.helpinghandcounselling.com
www.hypnoheal.co.uk
www.hypnotherapistregister.com
www.hypnotherapyforlondon.co.uk
www.noboundarieshypnosis.com
www.phobia-therapy.com

And for those who may prefer gentler methods, I would recommend

www.holistic-wellbeing.com

Acknowledgements

Like the Oscar acceptance speech for Best Newcomer (in a James Bond film, of course), I've played out imaginary book acknowledgements many times in my mind.

I'd like to thank:

My family, Marion, Arthur and Rob for their constant love and support.

Little Becky and Big (Stalingrad) Dave for their hospitality.

Fredd Culbertson, whose website phobialist.com helped start me off on this journey and provided much-needed information and inspiration.

Pom and Martin at Marshall Cavendish for the opportunity.

Abi and Dave (and Oscar and Molly) for the warm welcomes (and perhaps curing my Doraphobia?). Also additional thanks to Dave in his role as editor of *Fortean Times* for letting me reuse/rewrite material from my previous articles.

The one and only Mr Ej Zeida. The boy's a wonder, a wonder, I say!

Arwen Matthews, Emma Jack, Hayley Coleman, Lizzie Mathews, Natalie Cowell and Daniel Cardinal for their contributions.

An extra-special thanks to Ruth 'Rock Chick' Ratner for helping with the big words in the early days of list compiling (and for still loving *Hanoi Rocks*).

Tish for the loan of the camera that started this whole shebang.

The lovely ladies at the opticians; I *really* couldn't have done it without you.

Everyone at my kickboxing *dojo*.

Which must leave Si, *Sensei* and *Scooby Doo* expert and

'… *All ze girls* … etc.' sung in my best Julio Iglesias …

Word.

About the Author

Tim Weinberg is a freelance writer living in Brighton. After a long stretch in college, he embarked on a series of jobs from bookseller to night watchman without much joy.

Getting ordained online gave him the weirdness credentials he needed to become a contributor to *Fortean Times,* for which he's written about kung fu, clowns and Aleister Crowley. This is his first book.

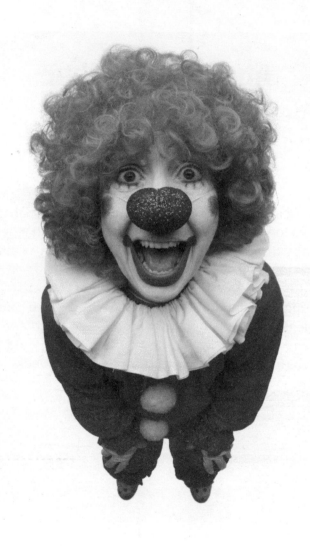